Journey Into the Unknown

A physician becomes a caregiver – and discovers God's strength to lead the way.

Arthur Sudan, M.D.

Copyright © 2021 by Arthur Sudan, M.D.

All rights reserved.

No portion of this book may be reproduced in any form without written permission from the publisher or author, except as permitted by U.S. copyright law.

Contents

Bad News	1
1. First Love	5
2. Alzheimer's – The Disease	10
3. The Formative Years	15
4. Learning to Suffer	21
5. Building a Family	27
6. Slipping	31
7. Faith Boosters	35
8. Mission Trips	40
9. An Active Life	46
10. Miracles	52
11. A Woman of Prayer	61
12. Living with Alzheimer's	66
13. Black Friday	72
14. Hard Decisions	77
15. Pulling Back	85
16. Downhill	90

17. Grace For the Journey	101
18. Caregiving	118
19. Full Time Care	129
20. A Little Help From Our Friends	137
21. Loneliness	143
22. Quite A Decade	157
23. Children's Perspective	168
24. Things I Never Thought I Would Do	182
25. The Move	194
26. Quarantine	217
27. From Their Lips	234
Continuing the Journey	250
Acknowledgements	253
About the Author	254
About the Book	255

Bad News

December 2008

It was just three days before Christmas and all of our kids were home for this year's holiday. That is no small feat when you have to coordinate four other families with your own and several grandkids to boot. And to make it even better, they were home for more than just the day, so we were really pumped about the time together. Once our kids started getting married, we got into a rhythm of Christmas together with our family and Thanksgiving with the in-laws one year and then the reverse of that the next year. Overall, that has worked out extremely well and of course this was our year for Christmas. Our family is very close and everyone gets along very well, including the spouses. We have lots of traditions around Christmas and as evangelical Christians, it is a special time anyway as we celebrate the birth of Jesus.

And so it was that day when my wife, Luana, and I came home from a doctor's appointment for her with everyone standing around and waiting for the news. No, it was not cancer. In many ways it was worse. She had just been diagnosed with early onset Alzheimer's disease. She was 53 years old at the time. Needless to say, the atmosphere in the room dropped like someone had let the air out of a balloon. Everyone began to cry and they started asking lots and lots of questions, most of which I had no answers. It was the beginning of a journey, and I knew more than anyone that this was to be a journey into the unknown.

So how did we get to this point? Let me take you back to the beginning, or at least what I think was the beginning. For the past several holidays the kids and I had noticed that Luana seemed more stressed than normal. This was very unusual for her as she is very chill and goes with the flow and does not let much bother her. She never needed things to be perfect and never minded when people would just drop by the house. That was indeed a good thing because we lived just a block down from our kid's high school and their friends would drop by all the time, with or without our kids. They felt very comfortable in our home as Luana was a gracious hostess, always welcoming and did not worry about the mess that was made. We didn't know why she was now stressed, but figured that she was getting older and maybe a little less flexible. Then during the year, I began to notice also that she would forget some things. It wasn't a lot but just enough to make me wonder. By the fall of that year (2007) I was becoming concerned, but I had not told anybody. We were at a wedding reception for the daughter of one of our friends and I remember talking to a doctor friend of mine who was also a medical missionary and telling him of my concerns. He discreetly laid his hands on her and prayed for her, which gave both of us peace. These memory lapses seemed to be worse during the holidays when she was most stressed and we attributed it to the stress. The kids were concerned because that Thanksgiving she messed up the recipe for one of the dishes we have had every Thanksgiving for years. But after my friend prayed for her and the holidays were over, things did seem to get better.

Luana is a nurse by trade but when she started having children, she became a stay-at-home mom and she loved it. She was a great mom. Then as the kids got older and were all in school, she began to do some part time nursing. She loved being a nurse and wanted to use her training. At one point she worked in an Ophthalmology office but by this time she was working in a wound care clinic. It was a nasty job with ugly, smelly ulcers and other wounds but these things did not bother her in the least. By February of that year (now 2008) I started noticing something new. The wound clinic closed at 5:00 but she routinely was not getting home until about 6:00. I asked her about it, and she said that she was just having to enter all of the data about the ulcers into the computer and it took her a while. Now Luana has never been very tech savvy, so if it was computer related, I could certainly understand. I didn't think much more about it for a while, but she kept getting home later and later. I asked her if the other nurses were getting home late as well. She told me that they all left right at 5:00. At the same time, I noticed that she was making a lot of mistakes with our financial program. She was the one paying the bills and would enter them into the program and at the end of each month I would get on and reconcile the statement. Again, since it was computer related, I thought it was just that but then I started putting two and two together. We thought the stress of the job was contributing so we decided that she should quit. When she did, she seemed to get better and things settled down for a few months.

But then it started happening again. The financial entering was getting worse, and finally, I had to take that over and just do it all myself. She started forgetting more things and I began to conclude that she really did have a problem and that it was not just stress. You see I am a physician, a specialist in the area of Internal Medicine, and we see lots and lots of people with dementia and specifically many with Alzheimer's disease. I knew what it looked like. The problem was that I had never seen anyone this young with it and that threw me off (to this day she is the youngest person I have ever seen with Alzheimer's, though there are certainly others out there with the disease who are even younger than she was). I did a simple MMSE (mini mental status exam) on her and she did not do well. So, I called my friend who is a neurologist and made the appointment for her to see him to confirm what by then I already knew. We did go in to see him and he did a similar mental status exam as well as a thorough neurological exam and pronounced the diagnosis – early onset Alzheimer's disease. That was the news I brought home that fateful day just before Christmas.

Chapter One

First Love

1974-1976

Luana and I met in the fall of 1974 at Baylor University while both of us were sophomores. Our stories as to how we got there are unique and certainly God-ordained. Baylor is a private university and is the largest Baptist university in the world. That said, it is still a small school with only about 10,000 students at that time. And neither of us would have been able to afford to go there if God had not intervened. We were both from the very middle of the middle class.

My journey toward college was fixed on the University of Texas as that is where my brother was attending and I had just assumed I would follow in his steps. But before my senior year in high school, I had a reawakening of my faith and began to get very involved at my church in Houston Texas, Willow Meadows Baptist Church. At that time, I also felt a calling to become a doctor. I did not know much about Baylor, but I knew people from my church that went there, I knew it was a Baptist university and I knew it had a very good pre-med program. So, I set my sights on Baylor without any thoughts on how I would pay for it. I often wonder what my parents thought about that idea (especially after I had my own children and paid for college tuition), but they never discouraged me from that goal. Two things happened over the ensuing year that paved the way for me to be able to go – both were scholarships. The first was related to my father's employment. He worked for Firestone Tire Company as a store manager for the wholesale distributorship in Houston. Every year they offered scholarships to children of their employees and there were only four or five across the US. My dad encouraged me to apply and I did. Part of the application process involved taking a test. I really didn't think much about it and soon forgot that I had applied (as you can see, I was very naive). The next scene, a few months later is forever etched in my mind. I was at school, at baseball practice, and I see from a distance that my mother is outside the fence and jumping up and down and waving a letter in her hand. My coach comes to tell me my mother needs to see me. I had no idea what this was about, but she had a letter from Firestone indicating that I had won one of the scholarships and it was worth $7,000. She was so excited and I was as well though not nearly as much as she was – to tell you the truth, I was a little embarrassed, as you might imagine, being a high school student.

The next had to do with another scholarship that I won. This one was a Jesse Jones scholarship and was through Houston ISD. I honestly cannot remember if I had applied for it or if they just awarded these to students based on their grades and community involvement. I went to Bellaire High School which at the time was one of the top high schools in all of the country. I was very blessed in that regard and I got a tremendous education. I finished with a >4.0 grade point and as such was considered as #1 in our class of 850 students (there were 18 of us who achieved that and I am not sure where I fit in those 18 but I was not the valedictorian). This second scholarship was for $3,000 which gave me $10,000 total. Today that would not even cover the tuition for one semester, but back then it covered all of my tuition, room and board, books, and a little spending money – for all four years! So, I was set and ready to realize my goal of attending Baylor.

Luana's father was a salesman for several companies but for most of his career, it was with Becton Dickenson. As such, he traveled a lot and was transferred a lot. She was born in Charleston, South Carolina, but had lived in New Orleans, Florida, New Jersey, and then finally made it to Dallas, Texas when she started high school. That was her family's last move. Her family joined Park Cities Baptist Church and Luana was very involved. When she started thinking about college, she really wanted to go to Baylor, but her dad thought that was an impossibility. Her sister who was two years older went to East Texas College and her dad, the wise man that he was, told Luana that he would pay as much as he did for her sister. Well, that was not even close to what it would take to go to Baylor. So Luana began to pray and to trust that God would provide a way if that was where He wanted her. Well, God answered that prayer by providing a scholarship through an anonymous person in her church. It was enough to get her there and she began applying. It was not until years later that we learned that the anonymous person was her Sunday School teacher. So, we both stepped onto the campus at Baylor University in the fall of 1973, but it was not until a year later that our paths crossed.

For that to happen, I have to confess that I acted a little like Jacob in the Bible, the trickster or the manipulator. I had seen her in the cafeteria and I thought she was really cute. I was with my roommate and I asked him if he knew her. It just so happens that he did. Here the story gets interesting. We all were a part of the Baptist Student Union and without knowing it, both Luana and I had signed up to be a part of backyard Bible clubs as a ministry through the BSU. Even more interesting was that my roommate just happened to be in charge of that program. He had made me a leader of one of the groups and I kindly asked him if he would assign Luana to my group. He did and our story begins, but I had no idea at the time that she already had a boyfriend, one she had dated for most of her freshman year. We began doing these Bible clubs with kids in the neighborhood and there, as I got to know Luana, I found out that she was not only a pretty girl but that she had an incredible heart for God and for people. I started falling for her, but I felt I could not act on it right away because I thought that it would not look good to the other members of our Bible club team. I still had no idea she was dating anyone (clueless), but fortunately for me, they were having problems and fighting a lot and she ended the relationship. Then right after the last club of the semester, I got the courage and asked her on a date. It was December 7 and we went to a Baylor vs University of Texas basketball game. That should have been an omen to her as to how important sports were to me.

After the game, we decided to just walk around the Baylor campus and talk. I was never very good at talking and was very nervous around girls. At the time, I was in the process of memorizing the Sermon on the Mount which is in the book of Matthew, chapters 5,6 and 7. I asked her if she would like to hear me practice reciting it to her. She was thinking that it was just the Beatitudes (which is just the first 8 verses) and she said yes. So, I proceeded to quote the whole thing and finished 45 minutes later. Amazingly she agreed later to go out on another date with me, but I do not recommend that for any other guy. I went home for Christmas a few weeks later, totally smitten and told my mother that I had found the girl I was going to marry. It was a good thing Luana did not know that.

She was not really interested in getting into another serious relationship, but we dated the whole next semester. It was somewhat comical in that at the same time I started pledging a service organization on campus called the Baylor Chamber of Commerce. It was an intense pledging period and part of what we did was to work generally till 1-2 AM (on projects around the campus) and I was also trying to do pre-med and I had to study a lot. Needless to say, I was always tired and sleepy. There were many nights that we did study dates (she was pre-nursing and she had to study a lot as well) in the student union building and I fell asleep. I am not sure what kept her coming back. For Valentine's Day, I had bought her a jade heart necklace which I gave to her along with a poem that I had written. The last line of the poem said, "And time only knows if our love will stand." She showed it to her roommate who started kidding her by telling her that I was in love with her. She countered with the thought that what I meant was spiritual love (that is not at all what I meant). That semester we also had the opportunity to be on the same team as a part of a much larger group of students from the BSU going to Malaysia over spring break on a mission trip. It was an amazing trip and once again I got to see her heart for people and her servant spirit.

Toward the end of that sophomore semester, we could see that the summer was approaching and we were going separate ways. In addition, she was going to nursing school which for Baylor was in Dallas and so would not be back on campus. We had a decision to make. Would we just say goodbye and be thankful for the fun times we had or was this a relationship we wanted to pursue, which would be difficult with the long distance. So, one beautiful day in May we went over to a grassy knoll near the marina and sat down and had a heart-to-heart talk. We discussed what we wanted in life, marriage, kids, work and so much more. It was amazing in that everything we wanted aligned perfectly. As individuals, we were as different as night and day, but our goals in life were as one. She remembers that day as the first time she really realized that she loved me. Of course, I had been in love with her for some time. We decided to continue our relationship, and that was a pivotal time in our lives.

Chapter Two

Alzheimer's – The Disease
2009

So, what exactly is Alzheimer's? Here is an excerpt from a blog I write:

> You may already know about Alzheimer's or you might be like so many of our friends when they found out about Luana's diagnosis. They said "I have trouble remembering people's names or I lose things. How do I know if I have Alzheimer's?" There is a lot written on this from a variety of sources and I will only give a decent overview, but from the perspective of a physician but also a spouse. Let me start by clarifying something that a lot of people get confused about. Dementia is the broad generic term for a problem with one's cognitive functioning (much like arthritis is a broad term to include many different disease states of the joints). It is a chronic problem, although there are some types that are treatable. Sudden confusional states are referred to as delirium. That is a whole other discussion and does not relate to our topic.

Alzheimer's is one type of dementia, the most common type, but it is dementia. However, not all cases of dementia are due to Alzheimer's. Other include Lewy body dementia, fronto-temporal dementia, prion diseases, normal pressure hydrocephalus, dementias due to thyroid disease or to B12 deficiency to name just a few. So when a patient presents with a complaint of memory problems (or more likely the family voices the complaint), the physician first must decide if the person has dementia. Then if so, he or she must try to determine the cause of the dementia. Unfortunately, it is not always a cut and dried diagnosis as there is no blood test like there is for diabetes. Compounding this is the fact that in normal aging we do lose some of our ability to retain new learning. The line between normal aging and dementia can be a very fine one. To truly diagnose dementia there must be defects in multiple areas of cognition. Certainly, the most common symptom is loss of short-term memory. But our cognitive skills involve many other functional areas such as reading, vocabulary, calculations, critical thinking, judgment, following multistep directions, long term memory, creative thinking just to name a few. If short term memory is the only problem then we will not give a diagnosis of dementia but usually call it mild cognitive impairment. It is like borderline diabetes. Many people with MCI will go on to develop dementia but many do not. The physician will take a thorough history (including the help of family members to find out what they have noticed) and do a physical exam to look for other causes of the problems. At this point he will perform a MMSE (mini mental status exam). This is an office procedure which takes about 5-10 minutes and involves a series of questions addressing different areas of cognition. The maximum score is 30 and below 27 is usually defined as dementia. Now it must be pointed out that a MMSE is not diagnostic nor is it very sensitive but it is a good helpful tool and specially to see how people are doing over time using repeated exams. Some people may have early dementia but a normal MMSE. There are other more sophisticated psychological tests that can be done to definitively diagnose these early cases and these are usually done by psychologists.Once the diagnosis is made then the next step is to do testing to rule out other causes of dementia besides Alzheimer's, particularly looking for the few treatable causes. This usually involves blood tests such as a CBC, chemistry profile, thyroid levels, B12 levels or sometimes others depending on the history which might suggest something else. Then usually a brain MRI is done again looking for other causes. If everything on exam and lab and MRI are normal then the diagnosis is likely Alzheimer's. We have always said that Alzheimer's disease is a diagnosis of exclusion and there is no definitive test for it. Practically speaking that is still true, but with the current research we can fairly certainly make a diagnosis. This is either with a PET scan using a specific type of dye or by doing a spinal tap to look at levels of certain proteins in the spinal fluid. The PET scan has actually been approved by Medicare but currently it does not pay for it. So, for the most part these are limited to research settings. To explore the possibilities of new medicines or other treatments, we did take Luana to Southwestern Medical Center in Dallas to the Memory Research Center which is one of 18 associated with the NIH. She has had a spinal tap and PET scans as well as multiple MRIs. Unfortunately, because it was a research project, we did not get to see the results.

When we do make the diagnosis of Alzheimer's, it is divided into early onset and late or normal onset Alzheimer's. The normal type usually begins after the age of 65 and age is the biggest predisposing factor with the risk doubling every 5 years after 65 until by the age of 85 roughly 1/3 of people have some degree of dementia. Early onset (EOAD) begins before the age of 65 and sometimes, as in Luana's case, well before 65. There are people who get the disease even earlier than she did at the age of 53, but as I said earlier, she is still the youngest I have seen.

The neurologist did do blood work and ruled out most of the other causes of dementia. At this point, we were left with a decision to make. He did start her on medication, but we talked about it and decided to go to the Memory Research Center in

Dallas. My main goal was to try to get her into a study looking at new treatment options because I knew that the ones we had were not very effective. The staff there were very professional, but also very compassionate. They did extensive testing (so much so that Luana cried because there were so many questions she could not answer). They agreed she had EOAD and with the treatment she was already on. Unfortunately, there were no available therapeutic trials going on at the time, so they just entered us into the database and saw her every 6 months. They took blood each time and did the neuropsychiatric testing. The blood was frozen and was sent all over the country to different labs doing Alzheimer's research and who needed blood samples of patients with Alzheimer's. In addition, they enrolled her into a radiological study looking at trying to diagnose Alzheimer's earlier and more definitively. This was the ADNI study (Alzheimer's Disease Neurological Imaging). It involved yearly MRIs, PET scans, and spinal taps and it proved to be very beneficial in its goals. This data which involved multiple centers yielded over 150 different scientific papers and I was proud that Luana was a part of that. But it did nothing to alter the course of her disease.

Chapter Three

The Formative Years
1976-1980

The next two years at Baylor then involved a long-distance relationship. She was at nursing school in Dallas and was back living at home, while I was still in Waco at the main campus and continuing my premed studies. We did our thing during the week and then spent most weekends together – either she came down to Waco or I drove up to Dallas. Fortunately, she was able to stay with her old roommate when she came and I was able to stay at her parents' house when I was up there. This was a time before cell phones and all we had were land lines. We could call "long distance", but it cost money for each minute so we would usually only talk by phone once or twice a week, and that not for very long. There was no text messaging, emails, or Marco Polo. We actually did something that seems so old fashioned now – we actually wrote letters to each other. I am glad we did, because we saved them and now can look back and read them. You can't really do that with texts or emails.

During the summers, we were even farther apart as I was back in Houston. That first summer I worked as an orderly in a hospital in the Medical Center to get some experience and to make sure that was what I really wanted to do. The second summer (after our junior year) I worked at a Seaman's center in Lake Jackson which was on the coast further south of Houston as a summer mission project working with sailors. In July, I took a long weekend and drove up to Dallas and met with her dad and asked for her hand in marriage and then popped the question to her. We then planned on a spring wedding right after we graduated.

Fortunately, I was accepted to Baylor College of Medicine in Houston in December, so the pressure was off for me and we could plan on moving to Houston for at least the next four years. The final year of school flew by as I was very involved in the university life as well as studying and trying to maintain a long-distance relationship. Luana was busy doing clinicals in nursing school and working part time. One event while she was there stands out as God's protection over her and later would prove to be a foundation building moment which allowed us to trust God when we really needed to do so.

She had finished a clinical rotation and was leaving the school at around 3:00. The school was not in the best part of town and a young girl should not have been walking there by herself. Luana is not a worrier and did not think much about it, even when three young men came up behind her and started asking questions. She is always friendly and trusting, so she was answering their questions until two of them moved in front of her to stop her. At that point, she realized that these guys were up to no good and she became frightened. Right at that time from across the street, a Hispanic man dressed in a security guard uniform called out to her to tell her to come over to him. She immediately ran to him and he explained that these guys were out to do her harm (sadly, a week later, another girl who was a student and a friend of ours was raped in the same area). He walked her to her car, and she made it home safely. As is typical for her, she wanted to do something nice for this man, so she made some cookies and the next day went to the parking headquarters and asked where the little Hispanic man was that helped her yesterday. They told her that there was no one who worked there that matched her description and furthermore, they did not even have anyone who worked the area where she was. She never found him so we do not know for sure what happened, but we firmly believe that he was an angel that God had sent to protect her.

One week after we graduated from Baylor, we were standing in the front of Ellis Chapel at Park Cities Baptist Church in Dallas, Texas reciting our vows to each other and uniting our lives with each other in marriage. It did not seem like a big deal then as I'm sure it doesn't to most all people who recite this vow, but it certainly did in our case. I think about it a lot now. Part of the vow says, "...to love her and cherish her... in sickness and in health." We were both young and totally healthy. Who thinks about it? But it is a big deal and even though I don't like it, now that I am in it, I want to honor that vow by loving and cherishing her even in her sickness.

While we are on the topic of vows, I know of a much younger couple who had to honor their vows. This was the son of one of my best friends at Baylor who had married a beautiful young girl he met at school at Samford University. They had moved to California where he went to law school at Pepperdine. He was about to graduate and they had just had a son when she had a hemorrhagic stroke. She required a 14-hour surgery just for survival and multiple other surgeries and procedures and physical therapy over the ensuing two years. He stood by her side the entire time and even now has to care for her. His willingness to abide by his vow was seriously challenged, but he was faithful and his faithfulness is a testimony to all of us. Now, 11 years later they have their own book about this, "Hope Heals", and their own ministry toward others with disabilities.

After the wedding, we had a honeymoon at a lodge in southwest Missouri on Table Rock Lake. It was a glorious time and a great start to our lives together. We then moved to Houston and rented our first apartment, which was a small one bedroom across the street from Rice University and less than a mile from the Texas Medical Center and Baylor College of Medicine. I began medical school and I loved it. I loved the learning, the studying, the skills training, the cadavers – all of it. Meanwhile, to actually make money so we could live, Luana began working in the surgical ICU at Methodist Hospital in the unit where the famed cardiovascular surgeon and trailblazer Michael DeBakey worked. It was exciting to say the least and she loved it and was very good at it. Unfortunately, the only shift she could get was the 3pm-11pm shift. This meant that she would go to work as I was coming home from school, and indeed we often met on the way, as we went through the beautiful grounds of Rice University. This was not a good recipe for newlyweds and after about 4 to 6 months she put in for a change and ended up on the 11pm-7am shift. It was better in that we actually did see each other, but it meant we did not get to sleep together five nights a week. Again, not a good thing, but she persevered, though she would cry almost every night before she left for work.

After working a year, while not being able to get changed to the day shift, she quit and went to work at a small private hospital on a med-surg unit. She was now on days and we were able to be together much more. In addition, the work was less stressful, and she was more relaxed and rested. Soon after that I was in clinicals which I loved even more, but then I was gone more than I had been. Toward the end of my third year in medical school Luana gave birth to our first child, a beautiful little girl we named Christy. At this point Luana went part time at work which meant that I would need to chip in for us to make it. As it turned out, I had accumulated enough hours that I was able to graduate nine months early. So, I went ahead and graduated and then had the fortune of securing a job as a research assistant for an infectious disease specialist at Baylor. My job was to be the doctor caring for the patients who were enrolled in our studies, testing new antibiotics. It was great as I learned how to be a doctor before I ever started my internship, and I learned a lot about antibiotics and infectious disease, and even learned a great deal about research. The great thing was that it was basically an 8 to 5 job, and I was able to spend time with Luana and Christy before I started my internship.

At this point in our lives, two things stand out as clear markers for what would define us as a couple and as foundational for building my character over the ensuing four decades. The first was our Sunday School class. We both grew up as Baptists and went to a Baptist church in college, so when we moved to Houston, we looked at Baptist churches and began attending South Main Baptist Church. It is a large church and like so many large churches, the best way to get involved and to know people is through a smaller unit such as Sunday School. We were fortunate in that the class we chose was taught by a couple named Sam and Susan Torn. They were about 7-8 years older than us and were an amazing couple. They led the class well with solid Bible teaching and fostered great fellowship which is what we needed at this stage in our lives. There were about 10-12 couples in the class and many of us are still friends these 40+ years later. We were all young and recently married and going through many of the same life events. In fact, when Luana got pregnant with our first child, she was one of 9 couples in the class that had a child that year. It was especially good for Luana to have those friendships while I was busy with school and then residency. It just so happened that the Torns became some of our closest friends over the years and we still keep in touch on a regular basis.

The second big thing was a medical school Bible study. Having gone to an undergraduate school like Baylor where there were Christians everywhere, I was a little apprehensive about medical school and how secular it would be. There were not a lot of believers, but we managed to find each other out and began a weekly Bible study. It was mostly medical students, but some residents as well, and spouses. We shared the duties of leading the group which was fine as we were all type A personalities. Frequently, we would split up with the women in one group and the men in another. I cannot overemphasize the importance of this group to my spiritual formation. These guys were all very smart (all doctors), all very opinionated and all committed to their faith. We were also brutally honest with each other. We would study a passage and you had better have studied up because if you did not give a sound answer, you got ripped to pieces (in love of course). This was when we met without the women who would never have let us do that. But it trained me to learn how to study the Bible and discern truth and to back up my position. This was truly a case of "iron sharpens iron." One person in particular stood out and he became my best friend and has remained so for over 40 years. His name was Dave Mabry and he went to MIT and loved sports like I did. In addition to the Bible study, we would play basketball and tennis and ping pong together. Both of us were extremely competitive as well. We would talk and share ideas and books and challenge each other to become better in whatever we did. He got married that first year of school and he and his wife lived a block from us and she and Luana became best friends also. They even had daughters born on the same day (our second and their first). These two things really provided a firm foundation for our marriage, our family and our faith and set us on a path that would carry us through even the toughest storms.

Chapter Four

Learning to Suffer

2009

During those first few years after the diagnosis, nothing looked different on the outside. Luana looked and acted the same and unless you were around her for an extended period of time, you would never know there was anything wrong. The first question was whether to keep it a secret or not. There are a lot of compelling reasons to do so and I do not fault those who want to do that. But for us there were two overriding reasons for letting it out. The first was that we did not want conversations to be awkward, wondering whether this person or that person knew. By telling, we could be up front with everyone. The second reason was that we wanted as many people as possible praying for her for healing and praying for me for the grace to care for her properly. And I can attest to the power of prayer in this, such that even though she never was healed, I was able to hold up far better than I ever would have thought possible. In fact, if only a small portion of the people who said they were praying for us actually did, then we would be in great shape. So, we told everyone – right from the get go. We were open and honest and did not try to hide anything. For Luana it was embarrassing as she felt less than whole, less valuable and that people would look down on her and treat her like an infant. But I was so proud of her as she was so brave. She did not let any of that slow her down.

But as I said, there are also legitimate reasons for not telling. Luana had already quit her job so that was not a problem. However, for those who are still working and especially those with early onset Alzheimer's disease, being honest about their diagnosis would almost assuredly cause them to lose their job. Even volunteer organizations may not want you working for fear of liability. In addition, if you had grandchildren, you might not want to tell for fear that your kids might not allow you to continue to babysit them. Obviously, as time goes on, you will have to tell for safety reasons. Then there are the friends, and you end up with a stigma and people treat you differently, which can be hard. I am sure there are other reasons and some very personal ones, but these are a few. Nevertheless, we chose the other route.

How do you go on and live a normal life when you have a diagnosis of Alzheimer's disease? It is difficult, but Luana did it about as well as anyone. She continued to stay involved in all of the things she had been doing – quilt group, Bible study group, book club, lifegroup, volunteering at Carenet Pregnancy Center and so forth. She continued her daily routine – got up and made her coffee and had her quiet time with Jesus and wrote in her journal. She continued to clean house, wash clothes, cook dinner. Most things she could still do well, though over time all of those changed.

But normal did not last long. They say bad things come in threes and for us it certainly did. The new year brought in 2009, and within four months I would have bypass surgery and my mother would have a disabling stroke. At this time, I was 53 years old and in excellent health. I had no medical problems, was on no medications, at normal weight, ran regularly (jogged would be a better term – I had run my first marathon just three years prior and had done several other half marathons) and played tennis once or twice a week. Toward the end of 2008, I began to notice chest pain when I would run or after a long hard point in tennis. To me, it sure seemed like what I thought angina would feel like, but I told myself that it could not possibly be my heart since I was the least likely person to have heart disease. I had no family history, did not smoke, did not have high blood pressure, did not have diabetes and my cholesterol was actually low. So, I ignored the pain and ran or played through it for about six months. By this time, I was beginning to think something really was wrong and I planned to talk to my friend who is a cardiologist. But our youngest daughter was studying abroad in Florence that semester and we had plans to travel to Italy and explore and meet up with her, so I put it off. We had a great time in Italy (ate too much gelato) and with our daughter. We even hiked up 2000 feet in the mountains overlooking the Cinque Terre. When I got home, I talked to my friend and he set me up for a catheterization the following Monday. I even ran three miles the Friday before just to make sure I was not over reacting. I was not. It was at this point that I told Luana. Needless to say, that did not go over well. I also had to call and tell my kids and they were not too happy with me either.

I felt certain that he would find something but that it would be one vessel and that he would put a stent into it and I would go home the next day and be back at work in a few days. Was I ever wrong? After the cath, he came in and showed me the pictures and all of the 90-99% blockages and told me I was going to have to have bypass surgery and would need six or seven bypasses. I was in shock as I could not believe what he was saying. There was no way that could be me. I began to cry right there on the cath table. I had always said that I would never undergo bypass surgery. But there was no time to think. He wanted it done the next day. We spent the rest of that day getting affairs in order (in case something happened and with a wife with Alzheimer's), calling friends and family, praying and explaining my actions to my kids. The next day they took me in and put in six bypasses. Fortunately, I was young and healthy and I recovered well – I was home in 4 days and after a week at home I was already doing more than the six-week rehab sheet they had given me. By 12 weeks I was back playing tennis and running, and by four months I went hiking to 11,000 feet in the North Cascades with our family and by December of that year (eight months after my bypass surgery) I ran a half marathon. Would you say that I was driven?

But I get ahead of myself – the other shoe was about to drop. Literally, the day I got home from the hospital, my mother called and was complaining of severe neck pain and could not move. It was not clear if she had fallen, but she was not thinking clearly. My son went over to her house and could not get her up and they called an ambulance and took her to the ER. She was admitted to the hospital and they did an extensive work up, but never really determined what had happened. But from that day forward, she was demented. It was obviously not Alzheimer's as it happened suddenly. I suspect she had a stroke. The CAT scan was negative but an MRI was not done. We tried later to do one as an outpatient, but she could not stay still, so it was cancelled. When she left the hospital, she came to live with us. My mother could walk and talk but she was confused and had delusions. At times she thought we were living in Alaska and at other times North Carolina. Somehow, she became convinced that I was operating a brothel and that Luana was one of my "girls." We tried showing her pictures of our wedding, but she was not convinced. She would take me aside and tell me that she could not believe that I would do this to our family. At times it was humorous, but as it continued, it became very tiring.

It was especially difficult for Luana, as now she had to care for another person and it limited how much she could get out or even babysit. This was important as over the three months after my surgery, we had two new grandchildren. In addition (and she never mentioned this) it had to have been hard for her to know she had Alzheimer's, and then every day watch my mother and wonder if that was what she was going to be like. We kept her for almost a year and then at that point I felt I could no longer continue to put Luana in that situation. So, with the blessing of my brother and sister, we put her in a nursing facility.

The first slap in the face of reality concerning the Alzheimer's diagnosis hit Luana shortly after my surgery. She had been working as a volunteer for Carenet Crisis Pregnancy Center. Shortly before my surgery, they had acquired an ultrasound machine for use there. These were critical, because when a pregnant woman sees her baby on the ultrasound images, she is much more likely to want to keep the baby. The center was looking for nurses to train to perform the ultrasound. Luana signed up for the training and it just happened to start the week after I got home. It was an intense course, lasting from 8-5 on Monday – Friday for two weeks. So, she left me at home to attend the training. I was skeptical as to whether she would be able to pass it, but I was not going to say no to her. It was so impressive and so like her that she was willing to take the course knowing that she had Alzheimer's. She always had a never give up attitude and it was never more evident than in that training. She would come home and tell me what she learned and try to study and get me to help her by explaining things. It was obvious that she was not picking it up well, but I kept trying to be encouraging. Unfortunately, at the end, they told her that she did not pass and would not be allowed to do the ultrasounds. She was devastated as she really thought she could do it. I was heartbroken for her, but knew that it was the right thing. I also knew that this was just the first of a long line of things she would not be able to do.

Needless to say, those six months from late 2008 to mid-2009 were not pleasant. But with the arrival of the grandchildren and my recovering well from my surgery and an incredible family vacation in the North Cascades in Washington, the bottom line for the year as a whole, was positive. Prior to that, we had lived a charmed life. I had not really experienced any setbacks or suffered in any way. I had often taught on the Biblical understanding of suffering, but it was all theological as I had never experienced it. But from this moment forward I could teach it from the heart, as I then knew it both intellectually and experientially.

Chapter Five

Building a Family
1980-1985

Those eight years in Houston (four in medical school, three in residency and one as chief resident) were pivotal years in our development as individuals and as a couple, but they also were a time when our family began to form. We got there as newlyweds with no children and left there with three children. Even before we had gotten engaged, we had talked about what we wanted in life and both of us wanted children, and we thought four would be a good number. Obviously, God is in control and we don't always get what we want, but we were in sync on this issue. After we had been married a couple of years, we felt like it was time to begin a family. It turns out that Luana was very fertile and she became pregnant on our first attempt. Her pregnancy was very uneventful and she gave birth to our firstborn, a girl we named Christy. We thought it might be on the same day as our nation's birthday but she held over one more day.

We had done the prenatal classes and I had been taught how to be her coach in the breathing. So, I was in the room with her and doing my part during each contraction, calling out "1,2,3, breathe". Luana was having nothing of it as she was in terrible pain (no epidural) and her arms were flailing and she was trying to hit anyone in reach. I am an avid tennis fan (I still play to this day) and every year at that time the biggest tennis tournament in the world – Wimbledon – is played in London. The finals usually end up around the Fourth of July, and that year it happened to fall on July 5th. In Luana's room was a small TV monitor and so while I was trying to coach her (and avoid her right hook), I was also watching the finals of Wimbledon. It was between Bjorn Borg and John McEnroe and it was an epic match. In fact, to this day many tennis experts consider it the best tennis match ever. I got somewhat distracted and while I was coaching, I would sometimes say "1,2,3, great shot!!" All of this was to no avail anyway as the baby did not progress and Luana ended up requiring a C section. Despite the 18 hours of labor, we were overjoyed to welcome Christy into the world, and to begin a journey for which we were woefully unprepared.

After Christy was born, Luana continued to work part time and Christy was in the day care there at the hospital where Luana was then working. As I mentioned earlier, I was working as a research assistant, but after the first year, I began my internship. About halfway into my internship year, I went with my former colleagues from the research lab to Chicago to present a paper. The night before we left, we went out to eat some famous Chicago pizza. I was unusually not hungry that night which was very surprising and made me wonder what was going on. The next day on the airplane I was feeling terrible but not sure what it was. I was looking so forward to getting home and letting Luana take care of me. But when I walked into our home, I found Luana lying on the couch as she was also sick. As I knelt down to talk to her, I looked at her eyes and they were yellow. I exclaimed to her, "Luana, your eyes are yellow. You have hepatitis!" Shortly thereafter I went into the bathroom to void and as I was washing my hands I looked into the mirror, and behold, my eyes were also yellow. We both got tested and found we had hepatitis A. We were in bed for a week and I was off of work for a month. Fortunately, my mother stepped up to the plate and took care of Christy while we were in bed. We did some tracing and realized that Christy had had some minor diarrhea off and on and that she'd probably gotten the hepatitis from the daycare and had given it to both of us. At that point, we decided to have Luana stay at home and not use the daycare.

One side note on that whole episode is that I had a friend who was a year behind me in training and was looking for an internship. He stayed with us for a night during his interview. He called us a few months later to catch up and report on where he was going for his training. He casually mentioned that he had recently recovered from a bout of hepatitis A. Luana and I looked at each other and we never said a word to him, but we knew that he had gotten it from Christy at the same time.

When Christy was about 18 months old, Luana began to get the bug for another child. We prayed about it and felt like the timing was right. Sure enough, Luana got pregnant the first cycle again. In years prior, once you had a C section you had to have one in all subsequent pregnancies. But by this time the incisions were different and they allowed women to have a trial of vaginal delivery. They gave Luana the option, but she wanted nothing to do with it. The 18 hours of labor were still firmly implanted in her memory. So, in November 1982 Luana gave birth to our second daughter, Amy. Though I was looking for my little boy, we were both delighted that we had another healthy child. Luana was a full-time mom and was great at it. Christy loved having a little sister and they became fast friends (as they are to this day). I was in my first year of residency, which was my second year of training.

We were not finished. When Amy was 21 months old (you can see a pattern), we started talking about another one. And yes, she conceived even before we had decided to try. We were in a tight race with time. By this time, I was the Chief Resident at Ben Taub General Hospital, the county hospital for Houston/Harris County. My contract ended at the end of June (as well as our insurance), and the child was due at the end of June.

Since she was a repeat C section, they were able to schedule her surgery for June 24th. She presented me with my first son whom we named Jason.

It was an absolutely crazy time as I had accepted a position with an Internal Medicine group in Waco, TX and we had already sold our house in Houston. So, after Jason was born, we stayed with my parents for about 10 days and then moved to Waco. My last day at work was June 30th and my start date in Waco was July 28th. There were so many moving parts over that month that it was hard to keep everything straight. It was an exciting time as new adventures awaited us, but at the same time it was sad to say goodbye to Houston. We had made so many good friends, had a wonderful church community and my parents lived there. On the other hand, this is where we felt God was leading us and we wanted to be right in the center of wherever that was.

Chapter Six
Slipping
Late 2009

By the middle of the summer, you could already see signs of her slipping. They were subtle but they were there and she recognized a lot of them. Here is an excerpt from her journal on 7/2/09:

> "Father let Jason be selected as a firefighter if that is your will encourage him. Father prepare Emily for a godly man let her meet him soon. Father, give the eye doctors wisdom in the procedure to remove the cataract in his eye. Let him not have any complications be with Jeannie, Debbie sister strengthen her with your love faith, and wisdom. Amen."

As you can see, the grammar and run on sentences were starting to show up, but her passion for the Lord and for people was just as strong as ever. Then we see some of her insecurities in an entry on 7/6/09:

> "Father, let the ladies at WIMA trust me to substitute for them."

This referred to her work as a nurse at my office. She would substitute for any of the other nurses who were out. She loved it and was very good with the patients and all of my staff loved her. Unfortunately, it was not the other nurses (ladies) who did not trust her. It was my senior partner who squelched any chance of her working any more in our clinic. I thought she still had enough mentally to do the work, but he disagreed. Mainly, he was concerned about the liability we would incur if something happened. I could see his point, but it was hard for me and it was even harder to have to tell her. It was just one more thing that she was not allowed to do – there would be many more to come.

When things like this happen, it starts to get into your head. Read this quote from an entry just a few days later (7/11/09):

> "Dear Lord, I know you love me. Forgive me if my pride has caused me to be afflicted with Alzheimer's. I repent of my sinful prideful ways. Please forgive me."

Certainly, this is not rational and intellectually she knew this was not theologically sound. But your mind can play tricks on you and you start to think crazy thoughts. The ironic thing is that anyone who knew Luana would agree that she didn't have a single prideful bone in her body. I never knew she had these thoughts as she never discussed them with me, and only now as I am reading her journal, do I see them. I wish she had confided in me so that I could have helped her.

"Father, I desperately need your grace, love and peace. Forgive me for my fears and pick me up from the 'Poor me syndrome'. Lord, encourage and strengthen Artie. Father, give him joy, peace, strength, patience, encouragement. Lord, please let me be his helpmeet and not his burden. Father, let Ginny (my sister) be willing to take Sara (my mother) for two months. Give me love and patience, joy and hope for Sara. Let me know how I can serve and love Artie better."

I never sensed that she was expressing a 'Poor me syndrome,' and if she did then she hid it well. She faced her Alzheimer's with amazing grace and acceptance, but refused to give into it either. She was not going to stop doing anything – we were going to have to take it away from her. As was typical for her, and really for most Alzheimer's patients, she had the fear of being a burden on anyone, but especially on me. Then, the reference to my mother and sister has to do with the fact that at this time my mother had had her stroke which left her with dementia, and was living with us. It was stressful in two ways. She was very agitated and thought that I was running a brothel and was always calling us out on this. But the other thing was that Luana was looking at this and realizing in the back of her mind that this is what she was going to be like in a few years. She never expressed that, but I knew she had to be thinking it. She needed a break and was hoping that my sister who lived in Houston could take her for a while. At the same time, Luana loved my mother and wanted to take good care of her. In the end, I took matters into my own hand and (with the approval of my sister and brother) placed my mother into a long-term care facility. It was an extremely difficult decision, as I had always told myself that I would not do that to a loved one. But I knew that I had to protect Luana from seeing that every day. In the long term, it turned out to be a good decision and paved the way for an even harder decision down the road.

When one has Alzheimer's, insecurities abound. This is seen in an excerpt from an entry she wrote on 7/26/09 (notice that all of these are from a one-month period of time).

> "Father, let the trip with the girls be good and not scare me with the driving and directions."

This was a trip to our lake house which was 90 miles from our home. I am not sure who the girls were that she was going with on this trip. This lake house had been in the family for over 20 years by this time and she/we had travelled there hundreds of times. That she was concerned, was an indication that things were worse than even I knew at this time. She was still driving to Dallas and taking care of young grandchildren when she wrote this.

What is so interesting about all of this, is how much insight she had into her own disease. I have many patients with Alzheimer's who are in such denial that even when much worse than Luana was at this time, would not admit that there was any problem. That was a beautiful thing. Luana never rebelled nor was she in denial. She confronted the disease head on. In retrospect, I realize that I was not much help as it was an incredibly stressful time for me. I was just four months post bypass surgery and still trying to play catch up at work, having missed a whole month. And I was trying to get my strength and energy back. My mother was living with us and driving us crazy. I had two new grandchildren in a six-week period of time. And added to all of that, my wife had a new diagnosis of Alzheimer's at age 53. That would be enough to drive anyone over the edge.

Chapter Seven

Faith Boosters

1985-1988

We never dreamed we would be back in Waco, but it turned out to be one of the best decisions we ever made. And that was long before the Fixer Upper, Chip and Jo, the Silos and Magnolia, and before Waco became a popular vacation destination site. It was small enough to where you could get anywhere in 15 minutes, but big enough to where you had most everything you needed. It helped to have a major university in the town, which brought with it plenty of sporting and artistic events. In addition, for me, the medical community was great. There were two hospitals but most everyone was on staff at both of them, and there was actually cooperation between the two (at least in the beginning). We had all of the major subspecialties, and there was a great camaraderie among the physicians. We enrolled our oldest as a kindergartener in the public school just down the street from our home and we joined the church we attended when we were in college. By now the college pastor was the main pastor, whom we knew well. We quickly made friends and jumped in serving in the church, teaching in the youth Sunday School.

There were two events in those first three years that helped us grow in our faith and changed our lives forever. My father-in-law retired toward the end of 1985 and he was looking forward to traveling with his wife of 42 years. Unfortunately, less than a year into his retirement, his wife (Luana's mother) started feeling bad and losing weight. A workup showed that she had lung cancer which was inoperable. She had been a heavy smoker all of her life, and would not quit despite all of our urging. She started on radiation therapy, but within four months of her diagnosis, the cancer eroded through a blood vessel and she hemorrhaged to death. This was incredibly traumatic for Luana, her sister, and her dad.

Luana was 32 at the time and had three young children. She needed her mother to talk to and ask questions, and to be a grandmother to our children. But she was no longer there. Even years later, I would catch her crying on occasion when something would trigger a memory, or when she felt like she needed to call and talk to her. It is ironic that our kids were roughly the same age when they "lost" their mother. They speak frequently of missing the ability to call and talk to her and ask advice, or to tell her something one of their kids did – something that only a grandma would want to know. It was a hole that could never be filled. As a guy, I could never really understand what it was like for her, and there was no way that I nor my father-in-law could make up the deficit. Later on, I realized that I could not make up the loss that my kids felt with Luana's disease. I did what I could in terms of babysitting, buying birthday and Christmas gifts and calling them on the phone. But that would never be enough. My mother was great and she loved Luana and they had a great relationship. She filled in as much as she could as well, but there is no one in the life of a girl like her mother.

That experience changed Luana in two major ways, and not in a bad way of turning from God and being angry all of the time. No, it drove Luana to a deeper, fuller relationship with the Father; she allowed Him to fill that void in her life. Her devotional times became even deeper and she related to Him on a more personal level. The other thing was that she became even more compassionate than she was before. She could empathize with other people's sufferings, and comforted them well.

The other event occurred the next year. As our son, Jason, turned two, Luana started to get the itch for another baby. We had always talked about having four kids, so we prayed about it and felt the Lord's blessing on it – so we went for it and sure enough she became pregnant. All of her pregnancies had been uneventful. Times were changing though, and for the first time with a pregnancy the OB doctor wanted to do this relatively new procedure – an ultrasound – as a routine investigation. She was about 20 months into her pregnancy, and when they were doing the procedure, the nurse doing it got very quiet and said that she needed to consult the doctor. Her regular doctor was out that afternoon, so she got his partner who looked at the ultrasound and confirmed the nurse's suspicion. He told Luana that it looked like the baby had hydrocephalus. This is often called "fluid on the brain" and it means that there is increased fluid in the ventricles of the brain, which then compresses the other brain structures and causes various degrees of brain damage. He said he wanted her to go to Southwestern Medical School in Dallas to have another US to look for any other associated abnormalities as they had a more sophisticated machine. He also told her something that stopped her in her tracks. He said that she needs to think about what she wanted to do as there were other "options." Of course, by that he meant abortion.

Several things happened somewhat simultaneously. First of all, we were shocked and devastated. I was not a pediatrician, but I knew enough to know that hydrocephalus was not a good thing. In situations like this it is easy for your mind to look down the road and think about how this would change every aspect of our lives. But this is also where we drew on the resources that we had around us and that we had developed over the years. We had seen God be faithful to us over the years, and had seen Him do the miraculous. Our faith in Him was solid. We also had a good support group in our Sunday School and our Bible study group. We went to them and asked them to pray for us and that gave us even more strength for the road ahead. Little did we know at this time that we would need this strength for an even more difficult and longer road that lay ahead.

Our prayers were twofold and based on the words of the famous trio, Shadrach, Meshach, and Abednego. We knew that God can and does heal, and so we were praying for healing for our little girl. But secondly, we knew that even if He did not heal, that we were going to love Him and trust Him, and so our prayer was that if He did not heal her, then would He give us the strength and grace to accept whatever and to be able to love and care for her.

The other decision had been made years ago. We were adamantly pro-life and the prospect of an abortion was not anything we even had to discuss. These are the kinds of decisions that need to be made before the event, since emotions then get in the way. We had a history with abortion in several different ways. We had a family member who had a back-alley abortion (before Roe v. Wade) and then died of complications. We had another family member who became pregnant while single and everyone around her was telling her to get an abortion. We pleaded with her to not go that way and she didn't and now has a wonderful child. Then in the first year of my practice, I had a young girl who came in and was pregnant as a single teenager. I had a long talk with her and was able to convince her to keep the child and she is now married and has other children and even grandchildren from this child that she decided to keep. Every time I see her in the office, I get goosebumps, thinking about what might have happened. The decision of Roe came down during my first year of college, and until then I had never even heard of abortion. At first, I thought it sounded reasonable, but as I talked with people and really looked into it, I realized that it was a horrible decision.

Well, the time came for Luana to go to Dallas to have the US. She checked in and they put her on a gurney where she waited in the hall before the procedure. While on that gurney, she felt the baby move for the very first time. While that did not signify anything specifically, Luana took that as a sign. As they were doing the ultrasound, they looked carefully and told her that everything looked perfectly normal. We were ecstatic. We called everyone who had been praying with the good news. It was a mixture of pure joy as well as humble gratitude. Why should God be so gracious to us, as there are plenty of babies who are not healed? Those are questions I cannot answer. As with anything like this that you cannot see, our joy was tempered a little until Mary Beth was born (the name was given as a joint family decision with Mary being the mother of Jesus and Elizabeth being the mother of John the Baptist, both born out of miracles). She was born and was a perfectly normal little baby girl. Here was another milestone of faith, another rock to be placed on an altar to God on which to worship Him. And it was another rock on which we would later need to stand.

Chapter Eight

Mission Trips

2010

The rest of the year was eventful in a lot of ways, and it also showed the character of Luana. Her prayer journal continually showed her concern about how to be a good caregiver for my mother. Here is one excerpt:

> "Dear Lord, I come to you today to ask forgiveness for my frustrations with Sara and the situation. Father, forgive me with my attitude that this is not fair. Forgive me for selfishness and self-pity. Lord, only you can give me the peace, love and joy to be the person you want me to be."

The situation with my mother was becoming more and more untenable, as she was so agitated and nothing would calm her down. But I had no idea how much stress it was causing Luana, and seeing her ask for grace to treat her better over and over again in reading her journals, was eye-opening. My other concern was the emotional impact on Luana at seeing what she might become. This culminated in a heart-to-heart talk about the future for Sara.

> "The talk with Artie about me, Sara and our future was difficult. I do not want to be a burden to anyone in my family. Please allow me to think clearly. Give me your peace, love, hope and joy. Father, give us clear direction to find a loving situation for Sara."

I then had "the discussion" with my brother and sister who were both in agreement about placing Mom in a nursing home.

She also repeatedly prayed that she would not be a burden to me and that she would love me well. Despite being rejected by CareNet to be able to do the ultrasounds, she held no grudges and continued to volunteer. Not many people would have the humility to do that. In those early days, she continued to babysit for our then, three grandchildren. And she continued to care for a lady for whom she had been caring for 17 years. She was mentally challenged and had two young adult children. Luana was her POA (Power of Attorney) and she was approximately our age, but had some medical issues and ended up passing away that year. In addition, she was volunteering for Meals On Wheels delivering meals to older people who needed help. She loved it and would write little notes of encouragement which she placed with each meal. She had a route with 6-8 clients each week, but often there were changes and it was in a part of town with which she was not familiar. Thus, finding each house for someone with dementia could be challenging.

> "Lord, let me be a blessing to the clients I see today. Help me find each home easily. Lord, give me your direction in every way."

Does that sound like a lady who had given up because of a diagnosis of Alzheimer's? No, that is a woman who lived life to the full with love and compassion.

In August of that year, we made a family vacation trip to the North Cascades National Park in Washington state. Our family loves hiking and loves the national parks system. With Luana's diagnosis, we thought this might be the last trip of its kind that we would be able to take with her. So, we were all in. I was able to find the perfect lodging for our whole crew online (which at the time was a fairly new option) and we even brought a friend to babysit the grandkids while we took some longer hikes. We had an absolutely splendid time. Fortunately, it did not turn out to be our last trip, but it shows the thinking we were going through when confronted with this kind of diagnosis. You never know how much time you have left.

In December we passed the one-year mark since her official diagnosis - without any celebrations. Then in January 2010, there was a major earthquake in Haiti. Our church has a disaster relief branch, and with the first week or so, we began sending teams to help with the relief effort. The early teams were focused on health care and in typical Luana fashion, she volunteered to go down and help as a nurse. It was a grueling time with a lot of heartache, as you can imagine. But there is one story told about Luana that sums up so much of who she is. This is told by Donny, who was the leader of that trip. He was called in to see this lady whose house, like so many, had been damaged and she had been hurt. In addition, she had breast cancer. She was sitting on the floor with her back to one of the surviving walls. There is no telling how long she had been there, and without food or water and certainly no attention to the wounds she had sustained.

Donny walked in and within a few feet he was met by this horrible odor, and he almost lost his meal. He immediately made some excuse and told her that he would be back. He went and found Luana and took her to the place. He left her there and then went and did some other things, but felt that he needed to go and check on the situation. He opened the door to the house and sees Luana sitting down beside this lady with her head on Luana's chest and Luana stroking her arm and singing softly to her. He was blown away by this picture of love in action. It was how he imagines Jesus with us, leaning into the filth of our sin and loving us anyway.

She was able to say yes to that trip because it was not the first time she had done something like that. Back at the end of 2003, a huge tsunami hit in the Indian Ocean between Indonesia and Sri Lanka and Thailand. It was devastating, wiping out whole villages and leaving the coastlines forever changed. Our church responded within the first few days, and put together two teams – one to Indonesia and the other to Sri Lanka. I had been on many mission trips all over the world, but I was not able to go so I encouraged Luana to go. She was a little nervous, but was always one to say yes to what the Lord wanted, even if it was out of her comfort zone. This one would be right up her alley as she was a wound care nurse at the time. I remember the excitement as we looked everywhere for medical supplies and medications for them to take with them. Several of us helped sorting them out and deciding what they would need.

Luana was on the team going to Indonesia and was with a doctor who was a good friend of mine, so I felt good about that. They were going to an area called Bande Ache. It was remote and with everything destroyed, I did not expect to hear back from them until they returned. A few days later, I was in my office seeing patients and get a page overhead to a phone call from our pastor. I thought that was odd as he never calls me. The first thing he said was that everything was okay. I was immediately confused since I had never thought that things were not okay. He then proceeded to tell me what he knew of the situation with Luana's team which had had a near-catastrophic accident.

When they got to Indonesia, it was a complete mess. There were planes from all over the world sending supplies and countless NGOs (non-government organizations) going to and from. The team wanted to get to the front lines and they kept asking people where they could best serve, and how would they get there. They finally settled on this village on the coast and the only way to get there was by boat. They arrived at the dock with all of their gear and they found this fishing boat (think Gilligan's Island). They managed to load all of the gear onto the boat and their team of 12 as well as the crew (and a few other Indonesians who happened to go along for the ride). They set out for what was to be a several-hour trip (again, as in Gilligan's Island, "a three-hour tour") when a fierce storm hit. The boat was being tossed up and down and everyone was soaked and was freezing. So, they ended up climbing into body bags in an attempt to stay warm. In addition, almost all of them were throwing up due to seasickness. I say most of them – but not all – as Luana was moving from person to person attending to their needs. They all feared that the ship was going down. Luana told me later that she kept repeating to herself the verse "For me to live is Christ and to die is gain." Finally, the captain got on the radio and called "mayday", the universal plea for help on the seas.

Sometime later, what appeared but a large Indonesian Naval vessel. They were able to get the fishing boat tied to the naval vessel and wanted everyone to climb aboard. The only problem was that they had to climb a rope ladder 20 feet straight up to get to the larger ship. This was as the boat was still being tossed in the waves and with pouring down rain. One of the Indonesians actually fell in and did not know how to swim so the captain had to jump in with a life preserver to rescue him. Everyone eventually made it and they were able to get into dry clothes and got some food. It turned out that the captain of the naval vessel was a Christian, which was very unusual in Indonesia. For them, he seemed like an angel.

By the next day, the storm had passed and the weather was beautiful. They got back down the rope into the fishing boat and set out for their destination. Unfortunately, their adventures were not over. It seems the tsunami had altered the coastline and the captain was confused about where to go, and they ended up getting stuck on a sandbar. They had to make a call and another boat came by and was able to pull them out. Eventually, they did make it to the village. All of this drama was just to get there. Once there it was worthwhile, as they attended to the many physical needs of the people, but also just listened to the stories of each person and who or what they had lost. There were lots of stories of the lives that they touched. It made a huge impression on Luana in so many different ways, but certainly gave her the confidence to step out way beyond her comfort zone, and know that God would be with her all of the way. It certainly made saying yes to Haiti so much easier. And I really think that it made her battle with Alzheimer's easier, for she knew that she did not need to fear. God was going to be right beside her every step.

Chapter Nine

An Active Life
1988-2005

We now had four kids. Our quiver was full. Since all four were C sections, we decided to have her tubes tied while they were in there. There would be no more babies for us. That stage of our lives was over. Luana loved the little baby stage, and in fact, whenever the youngest got about 18 months of age, she would get the urge for another one. She did get that urge when Mary Beth got that old, but there was nothing to do about it. Another interesting note about her tubes being tied was how freeing it was for her. She never told me this until afterwards, but she was always afraid that she would get pregnant before we wanted to. She had side effects from the BCP (birth control pill), and so she used a diaphragm. Fortunately, it worked pretty well.

We had already made the decision for Luana to stay home during this phase of our lives. We had done that after our second, Amy was born. It was not because she did not want to work – Luana loved nursing and she was very good at it. It was not financial, since at the time we were living just off of my resident salary (which I can assure you was not much). Of course, after I started private practice, the financial pressure was less. We did it because, after praying about it, we felt that it was the best thing for our children and our family. This was the best decision for us. I do not want to be judgmental toward anyone who chooses differently. This was not a popular decision even back then. Stay at home moms have it hard, and the society often looks down on them, as if they are not contributing. But Luana absolutely loved it and she was made for it.

Each stage has its own challenges. The baby stage comes with diapers (we used cloth diapers until the last one), car seats, sleepless nights, feedings and extra vigilance as to where they are. In a word it is physically exhausting. But it also has its rewards. There are the times of rocking and snuggling one to sleep, singing lullabies, watching them change overnight and learning new things almost daily. By the time Mary Beth came, Luana was in that mixed stage as the two oldest were now in elementary school. Luana did not waste any time. She immediately joined the PTA and soon found herself in charge of the annual school carnival. For our school, that was a big deal. It involved a lot of work and coordinating with a lot of other parents and volunteers. She actually did this multiple times over the 14 years that our kids were in this same elementary school. By the time our last one left the school, they were about ready to name a wing of the school in her honor. But that was not her only big event as she also was in charge of the annual talent show. This was the other big deal at our school and it also required a lot of work. Luana is not a natural or gifted leader. She is a much better worker, but there is no one who worked any harder than Luana did, and she was able to pull the events off in great fashion.

After elementary school (which was public), we did home school for sixth grade and then a small private school for junior high and high school (same campus). In fact, the elementary school and the private school backed up to each other and both were two blocks from our home so the kids could walk to school from K-12. So soon, Luana was involved in two PTA organizations. For the private school, she became the chairperson the annual garage sale which was a huge fundraiser for the school and was very important to the bottom line. Luana put in an enormous amount of work pulling this off, and she did it for many years, to the point where she became known as the garage sale woman. The last few years she even served on the board of the private school.

Homeschooling was not nearly as popular back then as it is now, and there were not nearly the excellent curricula and the enormous resources. And Luana was not thrilled about doing the homeschooling. We set it up where she would do most of it and I did the science. I took it seriously and taught it at a high level. The kids still complain about their sixth-grade science and how hard the tests were. On the other hand, they look back at their sixth-grade year with fond memories. They would work for an hour or two in the morning and then she would ask if they wanted to go and get a Diet Coke. Civics was mainly listening to Rush Limbaugh. But the time the kids had with Luana is a time they will treasure always. Fortunately, they learned enough to pass the test to get them into the private school.

School was not the only area in which Luana was involved. For most of the kid's childhood, we went to a Southern Baptist church. As with most Baptist churches, there was a solid culture of teaching and discipleship. This took many forms. The first was Sunday School which took place every Sunday either before or after the main worship service. Then, throughout the week there were programs such as GAs and RAs for the younger kids and then Acteens for the older ones. Then, there was Bible drill, a program to teach the books of the Bible and specific verses. Luana was a part of it all. She was the Acteen director for many years. This was a program to teach youth about missions both historically and practically. It was a weekly event and of course, required preparation. All of our kids took the Bible drill course and Luana was one of the volunteers. It is a great program and I highly recommend it. For many years, I had been teaching Sunday School in the 10th grade and after a number of years,

Luana joined me and she taught the girls, while I taught the boys. None of the girls probably remember what Luana taught them, but they remember Luana and how well she loved them. I have numerous testimonials as to how she impacted their lives. In fact, my nurse practitioner that works with me was one of those whom Luana taught and whose life she impacted.

The other teaching course she got into was a program called Precepts, and was a product of a gifted teacher named Kay Arthur. Luana was in the course, starting as soon as we moved to Waco. It was led by another doctor's wife who did a great job. After a few years, they moved away and she begged Luana to take up the mantle. Luana was very reluctant to do this as she is not a natural teacher, and does not like to get up in front of people (unlike her husband). But she prayed about it, and felt like it was the right thing to do. These were all ladies who were her peers and even older, some of whom were very smart. She was intimidated. Rather than run from the challenge, Luana put her whole being into this. She ended up teaching this course for 17 years. I can attest that whatever she lacked in Biblical knowledge, she more than made up for it in effort and in caring for the people. This is a very intense study and requires a lot of homework, even for the attendees. For Luana, it consisted of daily study and preparation. In fact, by the end, I was ready for her to be done with it, as it was consuming her. Even today, I hear stories from women who were in her Precepts classes and talk about what a great job she did. For her, it was more than the teaching. She loved those ladies and she ministered to them in the class and outside of the class. Her legacy lives long in the lives of those she taught.

As the kids got older and the youngest began school, Luana started getting back into nursing. She never worked full time, but did work part-time in several different areas. One of the first places she worked was at an Ophthalmologist's office with a doctor who was a friend of ours. She loved getting to use her nursing skills and loved the people and of course everyone loved her - both the patients and the staff. After that, she began to work part-time at our office when someone was out. The great thing was that she was never uppity as a doctor's wife, but wanted to be treated as just one of the staff. They loved when she filled in, as she did a great job and as always, the patients loved her. She continued to do this until she was no longer able, but she did begin a regular part-time job at the newly formed wound care clinic. They take care of chronic wounds that won't heal. It is a gruesome job as the wounds are often ugly and smell. This was really right up her alley, as she loved the hands-on part of nursing. She did this for a number of years and loved the camaraderie of the other nurses and staff.

One other area of nursing that she participated in was camp nursing. This was at Camp Ozark in the beautiful Arkansas Ozark Mountains. As a young married couple, we had gone there a number of times for family week. Then a friend of ours from Houston bought the camp and turned it into a Christian sports camp. For two weeks toward the end of July (always over my birthday), Luana took one and eventually all four kids to the camp, while she was one of the camp nurses. It was hard work but she loved it and loved being around the young kids and the young staff/counselors. Our kids absolutely loved the camp, and it was always a boost spiritually for them. She did this almost every summer for upward of 15 years. A bonus for her was that most of those times, her sister, also a nurse, joined her as one of the camp nurses. Then an extra special bonus was that one year (her last), she got to be camp nurse with our oldest daughter who was by this time also a nurse. As a testimony that life does seem to circle around, this past summer that same daughter was once again camp nurse, with four of her kids, and was to do it with her sister, also a nurse (but who ended up having to back out at the last moment).

As the kids got older and needed her less, she began to take up other activities. One of these was quilting. She had done some sewing since she was a teenager, and she made some clothes for the kids. Never one to be with idle hands, she then took up needlework. There are numerous projects that she did on the walls of our house as well as on those of the kids' homes. One lasting and enduring project was to do a Christmas stocking for each one in our family. These were intricate designs from a kit, with hundreds of little pieces and sequins, and took many months just to do one. When the grandkids came along, she began to do one for each of them as well. She did this until she could no longer master it. One interesting thing is to look at the last three or four of them and you can see the marked deterioration of the quality of her work as she got worse. But what she really loved the most was quilting. She was in one and sometimes two quilting groups, and each year a number of them would go down to Houston to the International Quilt Festival for a week – clearly the highlight of her year. One of the girls also had a home in Creed, CO and a group of them would drive up there for a week of quilting in the beautiful mountains. We have them all over our house and many of our extended family have one as well. One of her favorite statements related to quilting was that a person had to always make at least one mistake in sewing a quilt because no quilt is to be perfect, for only God is perfect. I am not sure of the authenticity of that quote, but it is so like Luana.

Chapter Ten

Miracles

2010

As the second decade of the 21st century began, life in the Sudan household was pretty much the same. Luana had passed the first year since her diagnosis (but it had been three years since her first symptoms) and on the outside, nothing much had changed. In a casual conversation, one would not notice that there was anything wrong. I would get comments like that from our friends all of the time. They would tell me that Luana looked so good (which she did) and thought she must be doing well. Those of us who spent any time with her knew differently. She was slipping. Apparently, I was getting frustrated with her a lot as her journal entries would indicate. Over and over, she would pray that I would not get frustrated with her and that she would not be a burden to me. As with most men, I was oblivious to that. I thought I was doing pretty well in keeping my emotions in check. But it is frustrating when they ask the same things over and over again, or when they lose things again and again. When people would talk about how well she was doing, I would get angry inside and want to shout that no, she is not doing well, and you should live with her and see what it is like. But I kept that all inside.

The course of Alzheimer's is different for each person but there are some typical patterns. Early on the curve is pretty flat with a very slow decline. After a few years, the curve starts to go down at a sharp angle and the decline is very rapid. Then depending on age and overall health, there is often another flattening where people have lost most all of their functioning, but do not decline much more and hang on for some time and often many years. In 2010 Luana was still on the flat part of the curve. How long one is on this flat part depends a lot on how early in the course it is diagnosed. We picked up on Luana pretty quickly, so she was fairly mild for a number of years. The medicines could have helped, but I am not convinced that they really do a whole lot.

With three grandchildren on the ground just two hours away, Luana spent much of those times going up and down I-35. In reading her journal, it seemed that she was going up there almost every other weekend. Adding to that was the fact that both mothers were nurses and were still working part time. Therefore, both grandmothers on each side were chipping in to watch the kids on the days they worked. It was good for my daughters and it was good for Luana and it was certainly good for the grandkids. In fact, the older grandkids still have some memory of Luana when she was more or less "normal." To complicate matters more, my oldest daughter, Christy, was pregnant with her third and had her at the end of July, a mere 13 months after number two. Then, my second daughter, Amy, also became pregnant with number two (born 10 days into 2011). So, there was a lot of action going on and Luana was able to keep up with it for the most part.

There were two things that concerned me in those days and for which I was super vigilant. One was whether she could watch the babies by herself. I had no doubt she could do all of the standard things, but was concerned about how she would respond if there was an emergency. The second thing was her driving to Dallas on I 35. It is treacherous at best and in those days, there was extensive construction. I worried about how she would do if there was a detour, or whether she would get lost or make a mistake and have a wreck. How long to allow a demented patient to drive is a very complex decision and there are no simple answers or formulas.

As far as how long to allow her to watch the kids by herself, I wanted the mothers to be the main driver of that decision. It was their children and I wanted them to feel comfortable with her watching them. On the other hand, they really wanted to believe that she could do it as it was free babysitting pretty much any time they needed it. Plus, none of us wanted to be the one to break the news to her.

Even though she was functioning pretty well, she knew that things were not okay.

> "Lord, I need your strength to not fall into the lies of Satan that I am of no value anymore. Cover that with your blood. Thank you."

> "Father, forgive me for fear of my future. Please give me your peace and a sound mind. Help me to walk with confidence that you will be my hope and peace."

> "Lord, each day let there be healing in my mind, and heal my Alzheimer's completely if that be your will. I love you."

> "Father, whenever I make a wrong turn or mistake, I get down and discouraged. Lord, help me to think clearly and not be a burden to my family."

One thing Luana never did was to deny the diagnosis or to pretend there was not a problem. She met it head-on. This is not true for all patients with Alzheimer's, and in fact, most are in some degree of denial. This makes it hard on everybody. That is one reason that I am in favor of being open and honest about the diagnosis with all of your family and friends, even from the very beginning. As you read her journal entries, you can see this and her concerns tended to fall into several broad categories.

The first thing was that she wanted healing from her disease. As evangelical Christians, we believe that healing can happen, but we also understand that it is not common and certainly not guaranteed. Luana was very realistic in this aspect. We asked people to pray for her and we as a family have prayed (and continue to pray) for healing. Early on, we went before the elders of our church and they laid hands on her but nothing happened. We do not give up hope or lose heart, and we are not mad at God. Our verse in this that we cling to is Daniel 3:17-18. The three young men are about to be thrown into the fiery furnace for not bowing down to the evil King Nebuchadnezzar. They tell him "the God we serve is able to save us from it and rescue us from your hand. But even if he does not, we want you to know that we will not serve your gods or worship your image." For us, we know and believe that God can heal, but that even if he does not, we will still honor and worship and serve him.

The second thing she often prayed for was to be able to think clearly so that she would be able to do the things she needed to do. Thirdly, she prayed that she would not be a burden to me or to her family. I think that if you polled every Alzheimer's patient, that would be at the top of everyone's list. We are an independent people and we do not want to be a burden. The other area of concern in her prayers had to do with her internal attitudes. When you start to lose your ability to think clearly, you become fearful of what the future might hold, you lose your sense of self-worth and value as a person and you can get depressed.

I am so thankful for her journal as we are able to get extraordinary insights into the mind of one in the early stages of Alzheimer's. This has been especially helpful for me, as she did not confide these thoughts to me, and I am only finding out now as I am reading the journals. It would have been helpful to know these things at the time, so I could help her better and minister to her needs in more specific ways. Hopefully, it will help others as they travel this journey into the unknown of Alzheimer's.

Shortly after these comments in May, my mother fell at the nursing home and broke her right hip. When we moved her to the nursing home, we had decided as a family (and not without a lot of soul searching) to stop the dialysis, which she had been doing three days a week for the prior six years, due to kidney failure from too much naproxen which she had been taking for her knee arthritis. Somewhat surprisingly, she didn't miss a beat off of the dialysis, so she survived. Normally, with a hip fracture the Orthopedic surgeons operate to repair it. But in order to do that, she would have had to go back on dialysis (so she could safely be put to sleep) and we did not want to do that. Amazingly, she had virtually no pain which made that decision a lot easier, and they were able to get her up and into a wheelchair. But hip fractures are often the harbinger of the end, and such was the case with Sara. Within two weeks she expired, most likely from a blood clot. It was the end of a very difficult chapter in her life, but as it was, we were thankful she did not linger in the condition she was in.

For most of the year, we had been planning on a trip to Uganda and in July it came to fruition. In 2007 a friend of mine and a fellow physician felt the call of God and moved with his wife to Uganda to begin an orphanage, a school and a hospital. I had been there with a team in 2008, and by now they were ready to begin some medical ventures. We formed a team from our

Lifegroup at church, with me as the physician and Luana and another lady as nurses, and then seven others as support personnel. We met regularly throughout the year to prepare ourselves medically and spiritually.

Uganda is not an easy place to get to, as you have two nine-hour flights – one to London and then the second to Entebbe (Uganda). You have to spend the night in Entebbe after you get there and then take a six-hour drive up north to the place, which is called Restoration Gateway. It basically takes about 48 hours and you are worn out by then. I was the leader of the team and thus I had the added stress of making sure that everyone got through all of the security and customs and had their passports. But this trip was doubly stressful as I had the added worry of Luana getting lost in one of the airports. Nevertheless, we made it without incident.

Restoration Gateway is on 500 acres in the northern part of Uganda, basically in the middle of nowhere. It sits right on the Nile River and really is beautiful. By this time, they had built several pods of orphan homes and had their first three orphans. There was no hospital yet, but they had purchased a large truck and had the side modified to be able to open up and to operate a medical clinic inside of it. We were to be the pioneers for this adventure. It was a bare-bones clinic, but we had brought a lot of medications and other supplies. We had no ability to do any lab work or X-rays. My friend had contacted some village leaders about hosting a clinic in their village. So, we drive this big truck further into the middle of nowhere and park it in a little clearing. Nobody was around, and I was thinking that this was insane and a total failure. But within an hour, as we were setting up, people started coming literally out of the woodwork (actually, grass fields), and before long, we had a huge crowd.

I was in the truck at a little card table and the nurses alternated between checking people in and taking vital signs and assisting me. One of our team served as the "pharmacist" and the others did crowd control and visited with the people and also prayed for many of them. We also had an interpreter with me. We probably saw 100 patients that day and it really worked well. Then, as the sun started to go down, we closed the clinic and the side door of the truck and used a white sheet as a screen for a movie. We showed the people who were there the Jesus Film in their own language. They loved it, and afterward, a local pastor shared the gospel and many people gave their lives to Christ. It was 10:00 at night by the time we got home, but it was a full and fun day. Luana did really well in her role as nurse – she was in her comfort zone. We did these clinics and movie night three times in the ten days we were there. The rest of the time, we helped the workers do some of the construction and just got to know and love on the people.

There are three events that happened on that trip that were really life-changing for us, and helped to prepare us for what was coming. As I mentioned, during the clinics some of our team were outside of the truck praying for people (for anything but specifically for healing), many of whom I had just seen and examined. One elderly man who had been deaf and dumb was prayed for and he began to hear for the first time in years, and started talking some, though not clearly. Our team was overjoyed and our faith was strengthened. Later that day another old man came with a bad limp and a makeshift cane which he used to get around. After prayer, the man's hip pain went away, and he left and gave the team members his cane (which they saved and brought back to the states). Again, a big faith booster.

The third event had to do with an old lady who they brought to me because she had not been able to walk for the past ten years. In fact, they literally carried her to see me. I spoke with her and the family and examined her briefly, but it was obvious that I was not going to be able to do anything to really help her. I sent her back out of the truck and spoke to our team to begin praying for her. I then saw a few other patients, and then we were going to break for lunch. I looked over and saw this lady with the team praying for her. At this point, I felt like I heard the Lord (in my mind) tell me to tell her to get up and walk. I politely replied to the Lord that if I did that then I could look very foolish. He then replied back to me that that was okay. He was not worried about me looking foolish – only about me being obedient. So, I took a deep breath and looked down on this lady who was sitting on the ground (I was still up in the truck). I called her name and she looked up at me and I calmly told her to get up and walk. Though she did not speak English, she obeyed and stood up and began to walk for the first time in years. Needless to say, I was blown away. I have always believed in healing, but this was the first person that I had seen healed in my presence. Now, I need to say that I do not normally hear these kinds of things from the Lord or have these conversations. Also, I did not pray for her healing – I commanded her to walk. This was the first and even to this day, the only time I have done that. That one event so strengthened my faith that it became another stone of remembrance that I put in my altar to God, and it has helped me immensely during the ensuing years in the struggle with Alzheimer's.

One other short story happened during this time which affected me deeply and which I could not understand at the time. Years later, when I was in a similar situation, it came back to me. I love hiking and still my favorite hike was my first one, Half Dome in Yosemite National Park. I did it first with my good friend from medical school, Dave Mabry, who I mentioned earlier. We did it by ourselves back in 1989. Then when our sons turned 16, we decided to do it again, this time with them. It was spectacular once again. As we were talking, I asked him how he was doing physically, since he had developed prostate cancer at the age of 45. He said that he was doing well and all of his checkups were normal. Then he said something that rocked my world. In the beginning, it was touch and go and he was not sure if he would be around to see his kids grow up. This caused him to push even deeper into the Lord. Then he told me that his relationship with God was so close that he almost wished the cancer would come back so he could go there again. I was blown away. I had never heard anything like that and I could not relate at all. Up to this point, I had not really suffered at all. But, boy was I about to find out first hand what that was all about.

Chapter Eleven

A Woman of Prayer
2006

Fortunately, Luana has always been a good journal writer, and we have kept all of them. I have been a lot more irregular in writing in a journal until the past few years. And of course, as we get older, all of our memories grow a little faded, so it helps to have her journals to supply any missing information in my own memories. I had not planned on reading through her journals until after she passed, but in preparing for writing this story, I needed the information locked away in these journals. I did give a few of them to my daughters to read and to be encouraged and to remember what an amazing woman she was. They have enjoyed having them.

As I read through them, a number of different themes emerged. Many of these came as a shock to me. Many I knew very well. One very surprising theme was how much she confessed her sins and prayed for forgiveness. Now, she was not very specific on these, and I have to wonder if this was just generalization, or if she really felt a burden of sin. I wonder this because Luana was the purest person I have ever known – both in her actions as well as her heart. It is possible that she had evil thoughts that I never knew about, but that would be totally out of her character. I think it was just her overall humility that caused her to write those comments.

Another theme that stands out is just how consistent she was in praying for people. She would not let go. There are prayers over and over again for people dealing with problems during specific seasons in life. You might see her praying almost daily for a situation for months on end. I can piece together our whole life based on what she prayed for. And it was a lot of different people each day, but especially those in her family.

One theme especially was how much she prayed for me. As I read, I was humbled, encouraged and challenged. One of her favorite lines was "behind every good doctor is a great nurse". I used to think that that meant a nurse working by my side, and certainly that is true. My nurse as I write this, Stinnitta, has been with me for 21 years and I could not have done all I have done without her. Unfortunately, she is retiring next month. But I really see that what Luana also meant that behind me was a woman of faith praying daily for me, and that gave me the strength to do my work at a high standard. She prayed for my work, my witness, my health and my teaching. One thing about me that she prayed, and that took me aback a little, was our relationship. Frequently she would write a prayer that she and I would connect better, communicate better or that I would not get upset with her. It goes to show how clueless we as guys can be. I had thought that our marriage was great. It was very good, but obviously, I had some issues I needed to work on.

Then there was her mind. Her diagnosis was in December 2008, but I first noticed symptoms as early as the fall of 2007. But Luana knew something was wrong in 2006. She never told me until later and it is so interesting to read her journals and see the struggle she was going through – and then to have to go it alone and not tell anyone. What a burden to bear. Of course, she was sharing it with the only one who could really understand and the only one who could actually help – the Lord. The earliest record I have of her mentioning it was April 26, 2006:

"Help me to think clearly and to do well at work."

A similar entry on 5/17/06:

"Help me to think clearly."

Then on Independence Day, 7/4/06 she wrote these words:

"Father, help my mind to clear up. Let me think clearly and remember. You are good. You are the healer."

Weeks later on my birthday, 7/30/06 she writes again:

"Help me to think clearly and reflect your love, grace and wisdom. Let me exercise my mind so that it becomes healthier."

Just a brief note in her post on 9/18/06:

"Give me your peace, wisdom and clarity in thinking today."

And the very next day she writes:

"Help my memory clear up."

Something that I would have noticed occurred on 10/9/06, but I probably did not think much about it as she was always disorganized. I could never figure out how she could do all that she did with such poor organizational skills. Another one of her quotes was that "organized people are just too lazy to get up and look for it."

> "Lord, help me to get my life more organized. Forgive me for missing/losing the electricity bill. Let me get my CM stuff done well. Help me to think clearly."

The holidays seemed to be a time when her memory and thinking got worse as it became a stressful time with the kids coming home and now with sons-in-law in tow. Thanksgiving was around the corner on this entry on 11/15/06:

> "Clear my mind. Let it think clearly like yours. Forgive me, Jesus, for a lack of discipline."

I cannot imagine the difficulty of dealing with this and not knowing what was happening. There is no mention in these early entries of her being concerned that it might be Alzheimer's, but it is certainly possible, as she had a strong family history. Both of her grandmothers and a couple of her aunts had it, so she knew there was a possibility. However, at this time she was only 51 years old and neither of us really understood about early-onset Alzheimer's. Her relatives were much older when they had it. I did not even know she was having problems, but certainly would never have thought about that at her age.

Whatever she was thinking, it was certainly bothering her a lot as she kept bringing it up before the Lord. It would be a whole other year before we would discuss it and two full years before her official diagnosis. And to add to the confusion/stress/joy going on, in October of that year we learned that our oldest daughter, Christy, was pregnant with our first grandchild. They had been trying for about 2 ½ years and had done pretty much the whole gamut – hormones, sperm counts, IUI (intrauterine insemination) - and were on the verge of IVF when Jordan (her husband) felt the Lord say to just put it all on pause. Then they get pregnant. This was another blessing from the Lord and another stone of remembrance in our altar. It seems so foreign, now five kids later, but at the time it was huge, and to this day when I see this grandson, I feel the goodness of God. As an aside, I do need to add that I would still feel that God is good even if He did not open her womb. I know there are many who have never been able to get pregnant and grieve over that. I do not begin to understand the whys, but my heart goes out to them and I have and still do pray for many of them.

Chapter Twelve

Living with Alzheimer's

2011

By now, we were in 2011 and were entering the third year of her illness. She was still doing pretty well. She was on two medications for Alzheimer's, which at the time was all that we had, and unfortunately still is. I am amazed that even with all of the money being poured into Alzheimer's research, there have been no new medicines or treatments for this disease in the past 15 years. The medications that are used do not make people better but help them to remain where they are for a longer period of time. Or, as we like to say, they flatten the curve. The first is donepezil (or one several others that act in a similar way) and the other is memantine. We know what they do in the body, but since we really do not understand the pathogenesis of Alzheimer's, we really don't know why they seem to work. Unfortunately, neither of them is very effective, and they only help for a few years before the inevitable decline begins. We kept her on them until she was near the bottom of the rapid downhill part of her course and it was obvious that they were no longer doing anything (if in fact they ever did). New medicines are desperately needed.

The other thing we were doing related to the disease was to continue to go to UT Southwestern Medical Center to the Memory Research Center every six months. This was a little hard for me since I went to Baylor Medical School and Southwestern was our chief rival. But it was much closer and we had family in Dallas, and when your wife is ill you will do pretty much anything. At first, we were just in their database, which meant that they would collect huge amounts of data on her (and other patients). That involved asking me what she was able to do and not do, doing a physical exam, doing extensive neuropsychiatric testing (which Luana hated as there were so many things she could not do and it would just make her cry) and blood work. They would then send her for an MRI. The data (including the blood which was frozen and stored) was shared with other MRCs over the country who were doing research on specific aspects of the disease. Periodically, we would be invited to participate in some type of study – it might be for a promising new drug, a vaccine or diagnostic approaches. We ended up participating in two of these. The first was the ADNI study which I have mentioned earlier and was an imagin study, and resulted in many important papers. I was very proud that Luana was a part of that. It involved an MRI every year, a PET scan, spinal taps and of course, more blood. Then we had the opportunity to join a treatment study. This was to look at giving IV gamma globulin which was done once a month for 18 months. Unfortunately, they stopped the study early because it was not effective (but it really didn't matter for Luana since when they uncovered the blinding in the study, we found that she was getting the placebo). That was the end of any other studies for us, and within a year of that, they told us that she was too far gone to be of any further use to them. That was a sucker punch and quite sobering. But they really didn't have to tell me, since I could already see it.

As I said, at this point she was still pretty active. She was in a book club and also in a Precepts Bible study (not leading anymore by this time). I would always laugh about the book club because she never finished a single one of the books, nor could she remember a single thing she read anyway. I cannot tell you how many times she would start the same book, not knowing that she had already done it. But she loved the ladies in it and they loved her and they were gracious to allow her to continue in it, and the fellowship was good for Luana. She volunteered at the Grace House which was an alcohol and drug rehab place for women run by our church, and continued to volunteer at Carenet, the crisis pregnancy ministry, as well as delivering meals through Meals On Wheels (though by this time she needed someone to go with her to help). She was also in a quilt group, which was the highlight of her week.

The year also saw two more arrows added to the ever-expanding quiver of grandchildren. We had Molly in early January and then my son joined the fray as his wife delivered another girl, Hallie, in August. Luana was still driving to Dallas and babysitting, which was occupying more and more of her time – which was totally fine with her – and me. Then we sent my youngest daughter, Mary Beth, to Uganda, to the same place we went the year before. She and a couple of friends spent about seven or eight months there serving the orphans, teaching in the school, hosting various groups coming for short-term trips, and loving on the women in the village. Before she left, she had begun to date a grad student at UT Southwestern Medical Center who was studying molecular genetics. They continued to communicate while she was away and then reconnected when she got back. By the end of the year, she was engaged and we were about to have our last wedding.

The wedding would not take place until May of 2012, but it revealed a hole in Luana's mental functioning that was much larger than I had thought. In all three of our other weddings, I was on the sidelines performing the three S duties of the father of the bride – show up, shell out and shut up. But this was different. Luana was not able to help plan the wedding. I had to step in and work with my daughter on all aspects – flowers, food, invitations, etc. Fortunately, my daughter knew what she wanted and we worked well together, but it is not what either of us would have wanted. It clearly marked the beginning of the decline.

Going through her journal for that year was also interesting. I could really tell some differences from the beginning of the year to the end. For one thing, her posts became less frequent. Often the entries were 3 or 4 days apart. They were also shorter and she began to make more mistakes. In August, when our granddaughter was born, she referred to her on consecutive days as Haley, Halley, and Halie. None of those was even correct as her name is Hallie. Also, she would get the dates confused. She would be in August, but then the next few posts she might write July and then back to August. Here is one post which was especially alarming:

> "Sept. 9th – Thursday. Dear Lord, this date 2008 our great contry was attacked by terroist. Lord I pray that those who have lost loved ones have run to you and given them hope joy love and peace."

Then this post in November illustrates more confusion on dates. My daughter, Amy has a birthday on November 3rd and her husband's is exactly a week later on the 10th. She gets this confused and in the same post, she talks about going through things in the attic to get rid of stuff, but cannot remember the word and calls it the garage ceiling. Our attic is in the house and we do not have a garage, only a carport.

> "Forgive me for not being organized to have a calendar (I should have made one for her) with their BDays Nov 3rd and 8th. Lord, help me with the task

that I have outside with the garage ceiling. Lord, help me get rid of stuff we don't need. Help me to think clearly and get my Precepts done."

And often the simplest of tasks were very difficult for her, and she would stress about it and was so worried that she would make mistakes. She was helping with a wedding shower for her friend and she was in charge of getting the invitations addressed and mailed. Normally that would be a pretty simple and straightforward task. Look at her thinking here:

"Please let me do a good job with the invites for Sarah's wedding (shower). I do not want to make a mistake. Lord, give me clear thinking and confidence as I make decisions."

That is an overriding theme for Luana and I think for most patients with Alzheimer's. Because they do not think well, they lose their confidence in anything they do. That then often leads to increased anxiety and even depression, though fortunately, it did not with Luana. This last entry I think summarizes what their mind feels like to them:

"Lord, please untangle the knots in my mind so that I may be clear for many years."

The year would also see us take several trips and Luana was able to handle them pretty well. In May we went to Charleston, SC which was special as it was her birthplace. It was one of the best vacations we have ever taken. It was very relaxing but we were able to do and see a lot of beauty as well as history. But I feel that we connected so well on that trip, partly because I was relaxed. I did have to be careful to watch where she was and make sure I did not put her in any situation where she might get lost. Then, in June we went to Omaha, NE to watch the College World Series. It had been a dream of mine for years and it was a blast. Luana did not care anything about baseball, but she was always willing to go along with me. Lastly, she was able to go on a girl's trip in December with her daughters and daughter-in-law to Chicago. I have no idea what went on there, but I can assure you that there was a lot of shopping.

Living with Alzheimer's Disease at this stage is a little like living with cancer. You are always wondering if it is going to come back. The difference is that with Alzheimer's, the question is not if but when your loved one will begin to deteriorate. Since everyone is different, there is no definite timetable and it can be nerve-wracking as you watch and try to determine if every "senior moment" is it. It can paralyze you into doing nothing and have you just crawl into your room and wither away. That was not Luana, nor was it my style. We were determined to live life as normally as possible. And so, we did. We traveled. She babysat. She volunteered and did so much more. But, by the end of the year, I knew that she was about to go down the steep part of the curve. I was prepared mentally, but was I prepared emotionally? I knew the end of this road and what it looked like, and frankly, it terrified me. I knew that I did not have it in me to do all that she would need in the future. However, I can honestly say that God has given me the grace to do all that I needed at the time. I have heard the statement (I do not know the source) that God gives us grace for the present but not grace for the imagination (of what the future might hold). That has truly been my experience. If I keep my mind focused on the present needs and not try to picture what the future looks like, then He gives me the grace to handle it. I have been amazed that I have been able to do things that I never thought I would be able to do.

Chapter Thirteen

Black Friday

2007-2008

For Luana, 2007 started out much like 2006. She continued to have times where she was concerned about her thinking, but there was still nothing obvious that I could see. That changed by the fall and for the first time I noticed some cognitive issues. At this point, I still was not thinking Alzheimer's, but was thinking that the stress of daily life was getting to her. I specifically remember discussing this with my dear friend and fellow physician, Tim McCall, as we were at a wedding for his niece. I told him my concerns during the reception, and he discreetly laid hands on her and prayed for her mind. That is my earliest memory of something being amiss. Then a few months later, the girls noticed that Luana was having a hard time with the recipes for all of the usual things she made each year. They too were concerned with her being stressed. But nothing else was mentioned and things seemed to settle down until the beginning of 2008. That is when things started heating up.

It turned out to be a busy year. In May, Luana and I celebrated our 30th anniversary and did a short trip to San Antonio and the River Walk. We delayed the real party until October when we travelled to Maui to take in the beautiful Hawaiian Islands. It was a fantastic time of walking the beaches, snorkeling, hiking the volcano, driving along the Hana coast, seeing Pearl Harbor and just being together. During all of this, she seemed relaxed and her usual self.

In June we had our very first Sudan family reunion as we gathered at Mo Ranch in the Texas hill country. My 85-year-old mother was delighted to have all of her children and grandchildren together. We had a wonderful time and Luana was her usual self and had no issues. One more stone of remembrance that happened there had to do with my nephew and his wife. They, too, had been trying to get pregnant without success. So, while we were all there, we gathered around her and laid hands on her and prayed (including Christy who was 8 months pregnant at the time). Just over a year later, she gave birth to a little baby girl.

Then, on July 2nd we welcomed our first grandchild into the world. His name was Jayden and the son of our oldest daughter, Christy, and her husband, Jordan. Luana was in another world. She took to grand mothering like a bear to honey. She spent the first two weeks with Christy in Dallas, and she was a huge help. As was so typical for her, she served them well (meals, laundry, cleaning) and was able to offer advice when asked, but was not a pushy grandmother. Her grandma's name is Mimi (mine is coach). And just six weeks later we celebrated the wedding of my son to his bride, Alex, with the wedding down in Clear Lake. It is so much easier to marry off a son than a daughter (and less expensive), but we did have to do the rehearsal dinner. Luana handled it all and she was really stressed with it, but I did not notice anything that made me suspicious that there was a problem.

Just a few days after the wedding, our joys were tempered by the news that my oldest brother had taken his own life. He had had a tough life but was doing well and was happily married (at least for him), but a few weeks earlier his wife left him and he was devastated. He was very private and did not let anyone know what he was feeling, so this took us all by surprise and we were in shock. We asked ourselves the usual why and what if questions, but of course there were no answers.

As 2007 rolled over into 2008, the situation began to get worse to the point where I knew something was wrong. Just the other day, I was reading her journal and I saw an entry in the very back of the journal that startled me. It was her reaction to the diagnosis.

> December 2008 "My Black Friday"
>
> "The Dx was made that I had Alzheimer's. I was devastated and ashamed even though it was not caused by me, other than a family 'gift'. Both sides of my parent's families had this disease. I had thoughts that I would rather have cancer and die than to be a burden to Artie and my family. However, our God is greater than our fears. God's grace is sufficient. I asked God to give me peace and He did. I asked the pastors of our church to pray for me, as well as all of our believing friends. This peace has remained. I never blamed God because we live in a fallen world and bad stuff happens. I am thankful I have had Jesus in my life for 42 years and He has always been my strength. I am thankful that we have a God who will never leave us or forsake us. Praise His holy name."

I am not sure exactly when this was written, but it was at least several weeks after the fact. There were several key points from this that I want to point out. The first was that she felt ashamed. Of course, she has no reason in the world to feel that way and she even knows it intellectually, but it still is a common feeling amongst Alzheimer's patients. Then, as the disease progresses, and they begin to forget more things, they feel even more ashamed. The second point was that she had thoughts that she would rather have cancer and die. She was a nurse and like me, knew what lay ahead. This was in no way an unreasonable thought. I have written elsewhere arguing that Alzheimer's is actually worse than cancer because there is seemingly no end. You lose the person, but you cannot grieve because they are still alive. Now, I am not really trying to argue – both diseases are bad and each individual case is unique – I was just making a point, and Luana certainly seemed to agree. The third thing is that Alzheimer's patients are horrified at the thought of being a burden on their family. Part of that is just our Western culture and the rugged individualism of Americans, such that no one wants to be a burden on anyone. But early on, most Alzheimer's patients have a pretty good idea of what the progression of the disease looks like, and they really don't want to be that person to their children (or spouse).

This essay also shows the deep faith that Luana had and which allowed her to face this crisis with grace and dignity. This faith, as I have tried to outline throughout this book did not just happen, but was cultivated over decades, so that when she needed to draw from that well, the water was deep. I have emphasized what I have been calling stones of remembrance where our faith has been tested and God has been faithful. In addition, she spent the first part of every morning with her Bible and a cup of coffee, reading the word and praying and writing in her journal. Then, there were years of teaching God's word through Precepts and 10th grade girls Sunday School. This faith did not just happen. She says that God is greater than our fears, and that He gave her peace. I can certainly testify to that, as she did not walk in fear, but had an uncanny sense of peace the whole time. She stood on the 42-year relationship she has had with Jesus, and the knowledge that He will never leave her or forsake her.

Chapter Fourteen

Hard Decisions

2012

2012 was the last year that she wrote in her journal, and even then, it was not nearly as regular, with a whole year in about a third of a small journal. The entries were shorter than the year before, and there were many more mistakes. By the end, she was just recording the day of the week and no actual date, so I am assuming she could not remember the dates. I lived through this and thus I know it but I cannot tell you how heartbreaking it has been to read through the journals and see how her mind had deteriorated. Equally difficult has been to read the agony she faced on a daily basis as she saw herself slipping. She kept praying that I would not get frustrated with her (which obviously meant that I was). I wish I could go back and treat her more gently and love her better and show more compassion to her. I realize that I was more focused on how her illness was affecting me rather than her own feelings and emotions.

This year marked the beginning of the really hard decisions of caring for a patient with Alzheimer's, and it came early in the year – toward the end of January. Up until this point, Luana had been driving to Dallas to babysit the grandkids on a frequent but irregular schedule. By this time, that consisted of six grandchildren in three families. At other times, they would leave the kids here but either way, she was doing it on her own. I knew that at some point it would have to stop. I was in close communication with all three moms, so that we could be on the watch for any clue that it was no longer safe. This was difficult as you can imagine and in many different ways. The first was that it would be hard to tell Luana that she could no longer do it. Secondly, it would be a big hindrance to the moms, since at that time two of them were still working part-time (as nurses) and the grandmas were the childcare. Then lastly, and really the most important, was the safety of the children. I don't remember the actual event that caused us to make the decision, but it was a joint decision, and here was Luana's reaction:

> "I came back on Thursday and I had the hardest day when Artie said I should not be alone with my grandchildren (I did not say alone, but that she would not be able to babysit them by herself). My heart was shattered. I could not believe those words. I have never done anything but to love them. Wow! God brought Amy to me and I quit the tears and we had a fun afternoon. I hate this condition. Give me peace and joy."

To her, this came out of the blue, but it was something we all knew was coming. And she was correct – she had done nothing but love them. She had done nothing wrong. What she could not understand (abstract thinking and reasoning are two forms of cognitive functioning that are lost in Alzheimer's) was why she was being "punished" without having done anything wrong. She could not see that we were trying to prevent any problems. The thing is that she could have taken great care of them for many more months without any problems – that is if there were no emergencies. The deal is that by this time, Luana would not have known what to do in an emergency – and that is the real key, and the tipping point in being able to babysit a child. It is a bit ironic in that as a nurse, Luana had always prided herself in thinking ahead as to what the worst thing that could happen would be, and then preparing for it in her mind.

Though I can't remember the events that caused us to make that decision, I remember well sitting across from her and telling her the news. The only description I can give was that it was gut-wrenching. She cried and cried and kept asking me what she did wrong. I tried to explain that she had done nothing wrong and that it was preventative, but her mind could not comprehend that concept. It was especially hard because this was the one thing she could do and do very well. It was like ripping out her heart. The interesting thing is that not long before this I had made an observation about her and the grandkids. By this time, she could not engage much in adult conversation as she could not follow the train of thought or think quickly enough to interject a comment. So, when we were all together, we would find her on the floor with the little ones while the adults were sitting around talking. The kids loved it since she was on their level and she gave them what few adults do – undivided attention.

This was the first of those major decisions. The others would come soon enough. You can no longer drive to Dallas by yourself. You can no longer drive at all. You can no longer stay at home by yourself. You can no longer be at home at all. Those were coming, but fortunately, there was time in between them to get over the trauma of the prior one. A few weeks later, she wrote this:

> "Dear Lord, as I sit here in this place, I feel like I have not done what I need for others. I have been so indulged in my own pity party that I have been selfish with my love for Artie as I should. He has blessed me in so many ways and I have resented

> him. Which is crazy he has been only good to me. Forgive me Lord, and I will ask for his forgiveness as well."

This illustrates another common thread in caregiving for Alzheimer's patients. That is the fact that they often lash out at the one who is closest to them, and ironically, the one who has been providing the most care. I didn't know she felt that way, and Luana never lashed out at me. That was just not in her character – even the Luana distorted by Alzheimer's. But I see it all of the time in my patients, and it can be very hurtful. Patients will say things they would never have said when they were well. As a caregiver, you know this intellectually, but it still hurts. You put so much time and effort into taking care of them, and this is your thanks.

As I mentioned earlier, my youngest daughter, Mary Beth, was about to get married in May and much of the winter and spring were spent getting ready for this event. Luana was just not able to be of much help and I stepped into that role – one for which I was totally unequipped, one that I did not really want but one that I had to do. Looking back, I realize that I left Luana out of most of the decision-making, as that was easier, and that I really should have let her participate in as much as she could. Here is an entry from her in March:

> "Father, I pray that I can have some role in Mary Beth's wedding. Lord, this can only be from you. I just feel not needed and I don't understand. I am unsure of who might not be invited. Let me know how to understand this without being sad. "

Looking at this now and seeing her hurt, I realize my error, but at the time I was working full time, trying to take care of Luana and trying to plan a wedding. Therefore, I did what was easiest for me – to just get it done – rather than to consider her feelings and take the extra time to talk it over with her and to invite her to the meetings or discussions. As we all know, hindsight is 20/20.

The wedding came off well. It was an outdoor wedding and on May 5th which should have been a nice day, but it was incredibly hot, reaching a high of 97 degrees. I had built a square arbor out of cedar branches we had cut, trimmed it in English Ivy and that is where the pastor (my son-in-law) and the bride and groom said their vows. All of the kids and in-laws were bridesmaids or groomsmen and the grandkids all participated as flower girls or ring bearers. It was quite a scene. Luana looked beautiful as the mother of the bride and was in heaven with all of her family there. I walked Mary Beth down the "aisle" to give away my last child. It was a sweet time but I remember thinking that with this, my work as a dad was finished. Sure, I would always be their dad, but no longer was I the main man in any of their lives and no longer was I the covering for them. It was a sobering moment. I am beginning to sound like George Banks in "Father of the Bride".

Less than four weeks after the wedding, we were blessed with our seventh grandchild and Christy's fourth child, another boy, named Barron. As always, Luana went up there to help Christy. It was bittersweet as she could not do nearly as much as she used to, but she could still entertain the little ones and that was helpful. And as was typical for Luana, she was always upbeat and encouraging to Christy.

In June, Luana and I went back to Omaha for the College World Series. By this time, I was having to be a lot more careful. I could leave her in the hotel room in the morning when I ran, but once we got to the stadium and surrounded by thousands of people, I had to be super vigilant. It was like having a child. I could not take my eyes off of her. What made it worse was that she could get super distracted and was no longer good at following me. I tend to walk faster than her, and usually, I would be ahead. Frequently, I would turn around expecting her to be there, and she had stopped or turned the wrong way. Therefore, I had to keep her in front of me or hold her hand. I could leave her in her seat while I went to get a drink or some food as fortunately, she was not a wanderer. Many patients will not see their loved one and start to wander off and look for them. It really makes a bad situation even harder. What was hard was when she needed to go to the bathroom. I would have to get up with her and show her the way, but then let her go in by herself. It was often agonizing, especially when crowded, when it would take a long time. I kept debating in my mind whether to ask a stranger lady to go in and look for her. Not here, but at other times I did have to resort to that.

Then, in September we took an amazing trip. We went with my brother, my sister and her husband to Europe. We had been doing some genealogy research on the Sudans and traced them back to a certain part of Switzerland. My brother was able to get in touch with a guy that did genealogy work on the side. His name just happened to be Sudan, and it turns out that we are distantly related. So, we decided to go to Switzerland and see the motherland and then tour other parts of Europe. I was a little worried as to how Luana would do. There would be lots of airports, plane trips, train rides, etc. That would be a lot of opportunity to get lost. But fortunately, on this trip, I would have three other people who knew and loved Luana who would be able to help me watch her – and a female who could take her to the bathroom.

It was a great trip. We flew into Geneva and then drove to the other side of Lake Geneva to the Gruyere region (where they make Gruyere cheese) where we stayed for several days. We met with our distant relative and he later did some research for us and traced us back to a John Baptiste Sudan in the early 1600s, and all of whom lived in villages in this area. It was pretty amazing. We toured a cheese and a Nestlé chocolate factory and hiked in the Swiss Alps. We then traveled by train to Vienna, Prague, and Berlin. Luana did great. She did not get lost (actually I was the only one to get lost which happened when I went on a long run in Vienna) and managed all of the daily changes without getting upset or any more confused.

The rest of the year was pretty quiet. There were no more babies, though by now Amy had one in the oven. Luana continued to go to Dallas to be with the grandkids (though now not by herself). Often our other sweet grandmothers on the other side, Alice and Cindy would take Luana with them when they would watch the kids. Or Luana would go up just to be with them, though not babysitting them. She also continued her volunteer work with Meals on Wheels (she would have to have a friend do it with her and several were sweet enough to help out), the Grace House rehab center for girls, and helping a blind lady whom she had befriended. She would go over and clean her home and then take her to lunch and then to buy her some groceries. She did this about once a month for many years. As things got worse, she could no longer do it by herself but she got her sister to take her and this continued well into 2015, to the point where her sister could not do the grocery store with a blind person and a demented one at the same time.

By this time, her journal entries were even less frequent and less coherent. Here is a typical one from December 2012 – no date was recorded:

> "Be the woman of God that loves Jesus Christ Lord
> let me do the correct thing for Arties Care Lord I
> make many mistakes and I don't want toto the

wrong thing to day. I love you and I thank you for your great love for me You are my supply and joy. Thank for the Frends that help me."

As you can see, it was getting bad and soon after this, she quit writing altogether. Her last entry was in January 2013 and here it is – again with no date:

"Dear Lord you are my light you are my hope and joy Thank you for allowing me to be your's You bring me peace and joy Lord I pray that our time with the Ogdens will be sweet and a joy Thank you for there life Lord thank you for there love for each other and the world."

From here on out my sources will have to be my memory, the memory of others, her sister's journal, my Christmas letters, and any other material until the beginning of my blog in 2015.

Chapter Fifteen

Pulling Back

2013

As we moved into 2013, life was about to present us with plenty of changes. I am not big on changes, so this presented me with a lot of challenges. Fortunately, most of the changes were good, though even some of the good ones were hard.

The biggest change for our lives was the relocation of two of our children to the frozen tundra of Michigan, specifically Ann Arbor. My son-in-law was a pastor of a church plant (from our home church here in Waco, Antioch Community Church) in Dallas and he had been feeling a calling to Detroit. At the same time, my son was also feeling a calling there. They went on an exploratory trip in 2012 and then made the decision to plant a church there and have spent the past few months raising up a team (as well as support). After advice from the board, they decided to plant the church in Ann Arbor so they could reach the university there and then later plant in Detroit. The actual move would not be until the end of the summer, but the pain of letting go was already in the works. It was really bittersweet, because we had always told our children that we wanted them to follow God to wherever He was leading, and we knew this was a possibility. But when it actually happens, it is hard to say goodbye. It was especially hard considering Luana's condition. She was clearly getting worse and not only was she not able to help them as much, but she was needing help. I was needing help in caring for her. This would mean that there would only be two kids living nearby and available to help. I discussed this with them in-depth, and I told them that I did not want for us (or any illness we might have) to prevent them from responding to the call of God. I meant it, but it was still hard to see them go. It was really hard on Luana because they were taking with them six (and soon to be seven) of our grandchildren. That was her life. It was the one thing she was still able to do well. She loved being with them and they loved her.

If you are keeping count, you probably deduced that this was also a big year of change in the numbers of grandchildren. We added three that year. In March, Amy gave birth to her third, a son named Burson, and then in July our son's wife, Alex, gave birth to her second daughter, Corrie. Christy was pregnant with her fifth child when she moved and she delivered a baby girl in December named Larkin. This was hard on them as well, since they no longer had easy access to free and experienced babysitters. We all flew into Michigan for Christmas and Christy entertained us all beginning two days after giving birth. She is a real pioneer woman. That is exactly what Luana would have done.

This year also saw another of the big blows to Luana. At the beginning of the year, Luana was still driving to Dallas by herself. She had not had any problems, but there was a lot of construction on I 35 and the potential for detours was high. She would not have been able to navigate a detour. In addition, I could tell that she was getting more and more nervous driving up there and you could even see it in her journals (I will say that during those days of construction, we all were a little stressed driving along those narrow lanes). So, I just decided that it was time to keep her from driving to Dallas. Interestingly, this move did not result in the flow of tears that the others did. I think that she was so stressed when she drove, that it was somewhat of a relief when I told her she could no longer do it.

The next blow was not long after that and I remember the circumstances well. She was volunteering at the Grace House on Tuesday nights and would then come back home. She had been doing this for years without incident. I even remember before she started, she wanted me to locate the house and show her which one it was and to write down the address and directions. Well, one Tuesday night I was at home and beginning to get worried because she was not yet home. Then, I get a call from Luana and she is lost and has no idea where she is. Luana has always been directionally challenged and did not have a good mental map of the city. I am talking to her on the phone and asking her to tell me the name of the street she is on. She was driving slowly and trying to find a street name. She then had trouble telling me or spelling the name. Finally, I got the name of one but I needed the cross street, and this was equally difficult. I told her to stay there and I got in my car and drove to meet her. I then had her follow me back home. It was scary as she was a long way from home and it was dark and I could not get her to really communicate where she was. This was before we had the "find your cell phone" app. Bingo – this was an easy decision – no more night driving. Luana did not push back on that either.

Before the two families left for Michigan, and in anticipation of that, we took a family trip to Lake Tahoe. I had heard many tales of the wonders and beauty of this lake but had never been there. So, we loaded all 19 of us onto a plane and flew to California, then rented three SUVs and drove to Lake Tahoe. It certainly is as beautiful as advertised. We rented three cabins in this one subdivision and right next to each other. It was the perfect setup, as there was space between them where we could all gather. During the day we did various activities – beach, hiking, shopping, fly fishing, etc. – and then at night we would get the kids in bed and we would build a campfire and the adults would sit around it and visit. It was one of the most relaxing vacations we have ever had. Luana loved it and did pretty well. Of course, she loved having all of her kids and grandkids together. Because there were plenty of us, I was not stressed, either in the airport or during the time at Tahoe. She was relaxed as she had no responsibilities, so that was also good.

Never one to give up, Luana continued to be as involved as ever. Obviously, she could not do much, but many of her friends stepped up to take her to events, help her and befriend her. She still did the Grace House as mentioned earlier, but I had to drive her. She volunteered at Meals on Wheels, but had to have another to help her and do the driving. She was still in the book club, but needed someone to take her and they did not care that she did not read the book. They still included her. She was in two Bible studies and again someone had to pick her up and take her, and again she could not really read the material or prepare for them, but her presence brought joy to the room. And as always, her favorite was quilt group. There were anywhere from 6-12 ladies in this group and they met in a little back house of one of the women. They did not all quilt – in fact most of them did not, but they did work on various sewing projects. Mostly though, they talked – and I do not say that in a condemning way but in a very positive way. This is good and needful for women. I think most women would benefit from a group like this.

It was so good for Luana when she was normal, but even more so as she got to where she could do less and less. At first, Luana did work on quilts (which was her favorite thing to do), but as time and the disease progressed, she was no longer able to do that and she switched to knitting. This was easier to do and at first, she could finish some projects, but with each passing year, she would start a project but not be able to finish it. Our house was littered with unfinished projects. One of her sweet quilting friends would come over to the house to help her finish some projects, but even that was not enough. Along with this, she would buy material (for quilts) and yarn (for knitting). Over time she accumulated quite a stash. The problem was that she could not remember that she had just bought something and then would buy it again. Eventually, she stopped even trying to work on a project, and then later stopped going to the group at all. When I started going through her sewing room (yes, she had a whole room dedicated to her projects), I found literally hundreds of rolls (is that what they are called?) of unused yarn. In addition, she had pieces of material in her closet that reached floor to ceiling over the whole closet. I had no idea she had bought so much stuff. Fortunately, my youngest daughter took after her in sewing talents and is incredibly creative, and has been able to use all of the material.

Chapter Sixteen

Downhill

2014

One of the hallmarks of dealing with Alzheimer's is change. A stroke can be devastating, but once it happens, the patient stabilizes and you learn to live with the new normal, Alzheimer's is a progressive downhill course. Thus, once you learn to live with a new normal, they get worse and you have to adjust all over again. This has been particularly hard on me as I am a planner and do not do well adjusting all of the time. I called the previous year the year of change, but more changes were certainly on their way.

Early in the year, I felt like the Lord was telling me that I needed to pull back and focus more on taking care of Luana. In fact, I felt like He said that in this new season, taking care of Luana would be my ministry. I cannot tell you how hard that was for me to hear. To give some perspective on this, I will give you a breakdown of what I was doing at the time. Kids were out of the house so that was not an issue, but I was still working full time. In addition, I taught a class on aging at Baylor University weekly (during the school year). I was leading our Lifegroup weekly and led a Bible study at the Manna House (which was a drug rehab facility), as well as a Bible study at my office every other week. I also played tennis a couple of times a week, jogged, planted a full vegetable garden, and did all of my own yard work, did woodworking projects (building my fourth crib), and volunteered (with Luana) in the nursery at church.

Fortunately, I am driven and have always had a lot of energy and a high capacity. I am not saying that I didn't need to slow down, only that it was hard. And these things were not burdensome to me – I really enjoyed all that I was doing. As I began to try to determine what to let go, I realized that so much of my identity and my self-worth was tied up in what I was doing. That is not good and I understand that now, but at the time I did not and was just buzzing along. The first things I gave up were leading Lifegroup and the work Bible study.

Luana's care was taking up more time, and I did need to devote more time and energy to her and to her care. Emotionally, it was difficult. I felt like the coach had pulled me from the game and I was just standing on the sidelines. I wanted to go back in, but was not able to do so. I knew intellectually that this was not the case, and that God can use us in many different ways. Still, it was how I felt. Nevertheless, I wanted to be obedient to what I felt the Lord was asking me to do more than doing what I wanted to do.

Also, during this time, another one of the big blows to Luana's independence happened. I decided that she could no longer drive at all. Here is how it came down. I was needing to replace a bulb in one of my tail lights. I was in the back of the car doing this, but I needed someone in the driver's seat flipping on the lights, turn signal and putting her foot on the brake. It was so frustrating in that I would call out for her to do one thing, but she would get totally confused and do the wrong one or could not locate the switch. At that moment, I knew that there is no way this person should be driving a car. At about the same time, my friend and insurance agent asked me about her driving and pointed out some statistics as to how people with Alzheimer's had the same number of accidents as people driving under the influence of alcohol. He then pointed out that I would have huge liability issues were she to have a wreck and hurt someone while driving with a diagnosis of Alzheimer's. That was sobering and had already gotten me to thinking that I needed to do something. Then, the Lord blessed me with the perfect opportunity. Her car quit working. It had about 220,000 miles on it, so that was not unexpected and I don't remember what the problem was, but it was not unrepairable. However, I saw this as my opportunity, so I did not get it fixed and it just sat in our carport. Occasionally, she would ask and I gave some lame excuse and she would then forget about it. Then one weekend when she was gone to Dallas, I called this ministry that took old cars and they came by to pick it up. She got home and never missed it and never asked about it until one day her sister pointed out to her that it was gone. All in all, that went well, and not many tears were shed.

Speaking of her sister, that was another blessing that came our way. She and her husband had just come out of working for a ministry called Athletes in Action and had moved to Dallas. After a few years there, she felt the Lord leading them to move to Waco so she could help me care for Luana. This was amazing, as they were obedient to move even before her husband had found a job here (he eventually did). She was so much help, as she would drive Luana where she needed to go and she would bring her over to her house (only a half-mile from our house) to spend the day. She started doing the Meals on Wheels with her and took her to the quilt group. She would also take her up to Dallas to see their aging dad and drop her off at one of the kids' homes to do her Mimi thing. This was so unexpected, but such a huge help to me. They continue to be to this day.

As Luana's condition deteriorated, her circle of friends did as well. I actually had predicted this and had seen it with my patients. I am not sure of all of the reasons for this, but I do have some thoughts. One is that people do not feel comfortable around Alzheimer's patients. This is not something with which they are familiar, and they do not know what to say or how to act, and it makes them feel uncomfortable. The easiest way to avoid this feeling is to avoid the person. Other reasons would include difficulty in communicating with the person. As time wore on, Luana was less and less able to make her thoughts known, and she became limited to short responses and very little spontaneous conversation. She did not really know any details of our lives or the kids which is crucial to any woman-to-woman interaction. Thus, get togethers were difficult and not mutually beneficial. It takes a special person to fight through that. It is one of the reasons that I tried to develop a friend list that I could call or email to set up lunches for her. I specifically encouraged them to bring along another person so that there would be some meaningful conversation. These started out well, but over time dwindled to nothing. Then, for some reason, with Luana housebound (did not drive and me at work) friends did not feel comfortable coming over to our house to visit her (I now know this to be a fact, because later when she went into a memory care facility, many of them went to visit her there).

When we talk about dementia and other neurodegenerative disorders, or even just elderly people in general, we talk about ADLs (activities of daily living) as a way of determining how much help is needed and whether they can live by themselves. There are five traditional ADLs – eating, dressing, bathing, going to the bathroom, and transferring. At this point, she was just beginning to lose those, and I will discuss each one in detail. But we also talk about instrumental ADLs – this list is not exhaustive but includes cooking, taking their medication, handling finances, and so forth. Luana was failing in several of those areas and I will describe them as I quote from my blog post. One was in the area of grocery shopping (quoted from my Alzheimer's journey blog):

"So why do you have 3 cases of Diet Coke?" I said to my wife the other day when she came home from a trip to the store with her sister. " I don't know. I thought I might need some" she said as we were putting them up next to the 3 other cases that were already there, as well as the bottle of coffee creamer that I put in the fridge next to the 4 other ones there. Grocery shopping is a necessary endeavor for all of us but it is especially challenging with an Alzheimer's spouse. Ours has been an adventure that has morphed over the past 6 years and I thought I would share some thoughts and insights that I never would have known, just by being a physician. First, you must understand that before all of this, I had probably been to the grocery store only a handful of times in my life. When Luana was first diagnosed, not a lot changed. She was still driving and went on her own. There were no major problems other than getting duplicates of things we already had and forgetting some items. But I could live with those as long as I did not have to do it. Later, we had to start resorting to a list that we would make together and I would leave it with her when I went to work in the morning. Two unforeseen problems emerged from this. The first is that she would frequently forget to take the list. The second which was really surprising and which I was totally unprepared for, was that she had difficulty even following the list even if she had it in her hand. Thus, she would come home without many items on the list and still with others not on the list that she thought we needed (because she could not remember what we had in the cabinet). The other interesting thing is that she got to where she would go to the store virtually every day to get a few items here and there. These were not things we had discussed but she decided on the spur of the moment that we needed, or for dinner that night. Part of that was my fault, in that we had a tough time coming up with a weekly menu for dinner so that our shopping would include what we needed. I was never a cook and could not think of meals that she could make (meals were always an adventure but that is another post). The other interesting aspect of all of this is that she wanted so much to be able to do things on her own since there was so much she could not do. She would resist my efforts to go to the store with her (not hard to do, as I did not want to go anyway).But alas, her driving days ended and so did her independent grocery shopping. Now, we make a list and go together (still not good at meal planning) and that works pretty well. She keeps wanting to put things in the cart that we already have, and she has trouble trusting me to know what is at home. The major problem now is that she will go with her sister when she goes to the store and for some reason feels like she has to get something too while she is there. That usually is something we already have at least one and often multiple copies of. The difficulty with this, as with most things in dealing with an Alzheimer's person, is that you have to balance having everything run smoothly and choking out her spirit vs letting things go and be kind of crazy but allowing her some semblance of independence/control/self-worth. That is a very difficult balance, and one we struggle with almost daily. I am a neat, organized person and it is easier for me to do things than to let her help, but it is crucial to let go of that, even if the end product is not perfect. God is working on me in that regard and has given me a lot of grace as I change. Have a Diet Coke - on me!!!

Another area that deteriorated during this time was her cooking. She was never a great cook (and she would admit it), but she had always cooked simple but tasty and well-balanced meals. But that changed, and it was a slow but definite downhill slide. Again, I will defer to a blog post where I have described it well.

One of the most interesting phenomena in our journey with Alzheimer's has taken place around meals. For most of our lives as a couple, I have worked and Luana stayed at home to raise the kids. As they got older, she used her nurse training and worked at a number of part-time jobs. But for the most part, she was at home and cooked all of our meals. I can make a mean omelet and beautiful pancakes, and can do the traditional "man meal" by grilling burgers or steaks. But outside of that, I am lost in the kitchen. Luana was diligent and always had well-balanced meals, but would be the first to tell you she was not a great cook and never really liked to cook. In fact, there is a sign in our kitchen (and is still there) that says "I kiss better than I cook". So that is the background when Alzheimer's took over. It is hard to know exactly when it changed, as it was slow and imperceptible. She wanted desperately to continue to cook (to maintain dignity and a sense of worth) and I let her. Fortunately, I have been pretty easy and have not required fancy meals, as long as my stomach got filled. One of the first things was that she was no longer able to follow a recipe. It seems pretty simple but it is virtually impossible for an Alzheimer's person to follow a multistep sequence of anything. So, that means she was left to cooking only things she already knew how to cook. That was fine until she was not able to remember how to cook the things she had always known. Thus, dishes had important ingredients left out or new things added which made for interesting tastes. Subsequently, dinners became much simpler and more bizarre. Often, I would come home to a meal of a chicken breast cooked in a microwave with nothing else. Vegetables became a thing of the past. Other times, she would cook spaghetti noodles and put them on the plate but with no meat or sauce. I tried to help out after I got home by adding some things, but she was very sensitive and got her feelings hurt easily. Often, she would ask in the middle of the meal if I liked it. Sometimes, to add variety to the meal, she would put out chips, or plain lettuce or uncut fruit. I could and did put up with that for a long time, in order to maintain her dignity. To make up for these meals, we would go out to eat 3-4 times a week, and fortunately, she did not mind, but that gets tiring. The real problem is what happened next. The straw that broke it was safety. I was worried when she cooked that she would set the house on fire, and I finally convinced her to wait until I got home before she started and that helped. We also bought a lot of frozen dinners which helped. Several times she heated something on the stovetop and forgot to turn it off. The same happened with the oven, and it eventually got to the point where she was unable to even know how to use the oven. But the worst was the microwave. Often, she would try to cook things in the microwave which were not designed to be cooked that way. Then, she would just put the thing to be heated directly on the round plastic plate that spins rather than in a dish. Then, of course, she had trouble setting the cooking times and really did not know how long to cook them. Finally, I had to step in and suggest that we cook together and not let her do it on her own. It was another crushing blow to her, as it was one more reminder of what she could not do. There were lots of tears, but she has now accepted it well and I do most of the cooking (if you can really call it that). These are simple things that you do not usually think about and come on so gradually that you do not know it has hit you until it does. But, it also emphasizes the importance of allowing the Alzheimer's person to do as much as they can for as long as it is safe, and even then, to forge compromises and not just take everything away. It often is easier to just do things yourself, but you really need to let them help.

We did get to take some trips that year. A friend of ours' daughter was getting married in Nashville. We had never been, so we took the opportunity to go a few days early and tour the city. We had a splendid time as we visited Vanderbilt, downtown with a tour of the Grand Ole Opry, the Andrew Jackson home site and more. Luana did well, as we had no schedule and it was very relaxed and we were not in any big crowds. I did notice that she got more tired walking than she used to, so we had to limit what we did or take more breaks.

Then in July, we went back to Uganda. This time it was just the two of us, and I was really nervous as to how she would do and if I could get her through the airports and security (and bathrooms). By this time, they had built a medical/dental clinic and I was going to work there and see patients. Luana was going to help as a nurse (at least that is what she thought – I knew she would not be able to do much of anything). We got to Uganda without incident and then spent the night in a hotel near the airport. The next day, our driver picked us up at the hotel and we began the long five-hour drive to Restoration Gateway. We were still about two hours away, and literally in the middle of nowhere, when Luana began to get very dizzy and nauseated. She actually threw up once. And then she totally passed out. I thought she had arrested as I could not feel a pulse. We were in the middle seat of a van and I had the driver stop and I laid her down with the thought of having to do CPR. I was also thinking what in the world I was going to do as we were hours from any kind of medical facility and there was no 911 to call. Fortunately, she began to breathe and I was able to get a pulse, though slow. She gradually began to wake up, and I got some water down her. We got going again and finally made it to our destination, but that was one of the scariest moments – mostly because of the desolation of where it happened. We never did figure out exactly what happened then, and interestingly, she has had 3-5 more of these spells over the years. We have done a limited workup and never found an answer. Because of her underlying disease, I did not want to do an exhaustive workup.

Other than that, the trip went great. I got to work in the clinic each day and see actual patients, and we had some limited lab studies we could do and some limited medications. It was a lot closer to real medicine than the bush clinics we ran two years ago. Luana stayed with me the whole time, and did not really do any nursing except take a few BP readings. She spent a lot of time holding little kids (right up her alley) while I was seeing the mother. We got to spend some good time with our friends that run the place, and to give them some fellowship and a lot of encouragement.

The last trip was back to Ann Arbor for Thanksgiving. All 20 of us gathered there and had a wonderful time – at least in the beginning. One of the grandkids, as it turns out, was sick with a GI bug when he got on the plane and before it was all said and done, 17 of us contracted the virus. Fortunately, it was only a 24-hour bug so we were still able to do most things. We got to experience snow, which was fun for the kids, and to cut down their Christmas trees at a real tree farm. And we got to do our annual Christmas cookie decorating contest.

The year 2014 was the first year since 2008 that we did not have a new baby born into the family. But 2015 was going to make up for that, as Mary Beth was pregnant with her first and Amy with her fourth. Later Alex, my daughter-in-law, would become pregnant with her third.

Chapter Seventeen

Grace For the Journey

2015

At this point in our journey, I began to write a blog about our story. I wish I had started it the minute she was diagnosed, so that the story would be complete. I journaled off and on (I am much more consistent now), but even when I did, I did not really write a lot about what was going on with me emotionally or with our relationship. Thus, my journals didn't help much. As we have seen, Luana's did and they have really helped to supplement my memories. In addition, they give an account of her thoughts and feelings which have been priceless. But from here on out, this will be all from my perspective, as she was no longer journaling and could not really express herself. Here is an excerpt from my first post explaining how it came to be. The date for this was 1/4/15:

> My name is Artie and my wife has Alzheimer's disease. That is not particularly newsworthy. I am also a physician in Internal Medicine and have been taking care of Alzheimer's patients for 30 years. That narrows it down a bit, but still, I am sure there are many in that category. My wife was diagnosed at an early age - 53 - which puts me in a much

smaller group. We are now 6 years into this journey. So why am I now just starting a blog on this? There are many reasons but a few stand out. One is that just this week I diagnosed 2 new people at a fairly young age with Alzheimer's, and it has been on my mind and I wanted to offer them more than just the usual doctor advice. Secondly, I was having my quiet time yesterday morning and was reading in Romans chapter one, where Paul was thankful that the Roman's faith was known throughout the world. So, I thought "what makes one's faith known throughout the world?" The answer is a faith that is in action and changes the culture around it. So, then I thought "how can my faith take such action?" I started to think of all the things I could get involved in, and then remembered that the Lord had told me this past year that my ministry in this season was going to be in how I cared for my wife. It would be hard and it would not be glamorous. But how would that affect the world? Then I felt like the Lord said to share it in a blog and He would do the rest. For those of you who do not believe the Christian faith, don't click out, as what I will say in these posts will cut through all gender, religious, cultural or racial barriers.

At this point, life was getting more and more difficult. I was having to take on more and more of the responsibilities of daily life, and as we will see shortly, responsibilities for Luana's personal care. When this happens, you realize just how much of the load that Luana had carried. I was a busy man and had a lot of other interests as I outlined earlier. None of that would have been possible without a wife who was supportive and capable. As much as Luana was changing, I was changing as well, and interestingly, for the better.

When you go through trials, you can take one of two paths. One would be to get mad at God, angry at the world, and be bitter and depressed. The other would be to turn to God for strength and support. I chose the latter and as metal is purified by the furnace, so men are purified by suffering. I never thought to blame God for any of this, and I knew that my only hope was to turn full face to Him and allow Him to work His grace in me. This was not a spur-of-the-moment decision, but as I hope you have seen throughout this book, it took place over a lifetime of seeing God work in the lives of Luana and me and walking out in faith. It took place in those daily morning times spent in prayer and worship of God, even when I was tired and felt nothing. It took place in those events that I have referred to as stones of remembrance with which to build my altar to God.

I do not want to make this super-spiritual. It was hard and I shed a lot of tears. But God has proven faithful and has worked His sanctifying grace in my life. I am a better man than I was before this disease. I often lament that it took this for me to be open enough for God to be able to do His work in me. These changes I see in myself are from my perspective, but I have shared it enough with other people who have seen the changes and would agree. I am much more patient now with other people and situations. I am more compassionate with people (though still nowhere near like Luana was) and more sensitive to their needs. I do not get angry nearly as much. I am gentler in dealing with others and I have an inner peace in my life. If this sounds like the fruit of the Spirit, then that is precisely what He is producing in me. No, I have not arrived – only that in all of these things, I am better now than I was before. This is part of the reason that when people ask how I am doing, I can honestly say that I feel incredibly blessed. The other part is that I have four wonderful children and (at this point) 13 grandchildren, a good job, great friends and good health.

The other aspect to the spiritual side of this journey, is just how faithful God has been to give me what I need. I have said repeatedly that because of my work and having seen so many patients at all points in the Alzheimer's spectrum, I knew what the end was going to look like, and it terrified me. If I allowed myself to even imagine the point where she is now (as I write this book), I would have decompensated. But I knew that I could not go there. It was not healthy. I had to literally take it a day at a time. I could not imagine doing what it takes now to care for her, when we first started. I did not think I had it in me. But God does not give us grace for the imagination – He gives us grace for the day. Over the past seven years of her disease, He has given me the grace to do the next step. He has given me the grace to be patient with her. He has given me the grace to step in and do the cooking and the laundry. He has given me the grace to pick out her clothes and help her get dressed in the mornings. Now, I am not as fearful of what lies ahead, because I know that the same God who has given me the grace to do what needed to be done today, will give me the grace to do what needs to be done tomorrow. I still catch myself looking ahead and it is still scary, but I don't stay there. I say all of this only to encourage others who may be on a similar journey with Alzheimer's, or any other form of trial or suffering. There is a book on this topic that I would recommend called <u>Beautiful Battlefields</u> by Bo Stearns.

As usual, we made some trips this year. In May we went to Michigan to see the kids up there and it was a great time. That is a beautiful time of year in Michigan. Then, in June we all met halfway in southeastern Missouri at a small, secluded place on a creek and with a pond and lots of room to roam. It was incredibly relaxing. There was plenty to do – hiking, rafting, swimming in the creek – but also time to just sit and visit outside while the kids played. These times were good for our family as we got to spend time with each other, encourage one another, allow the cousins to play with each other and develop those relationships and build up a whole scrapbook of memories. But it was good also for Luana to be in a situation where she could be a part, but did not have to do anything and where she was surrounded by people she loved and who loved her. It was good for me, as I had plenty of help. But it was also good for the grandkids, as they got to see Mimi and be loved by her, but they also got to see that everyone is not always perfect and whole. They got to see how we as her family treated her with honor and respect and invited her to be a part in spite of her limitations. Later we went back to Michigan in October to meet the newest granddaughter, born to Alex and Jason.

Speaking of which, this year was a spectacular year in that we welcomed three new grandchildren into the world. We had a similar year in 2013. March brought us the first child of Mary Beth and Alejandro, a girl named Sundance (not to be confused with a dog we had by that name when the kids were young). Then in July, Amy gave birth to her fourth child, another girl named Lucy. Of note is that Amy's family perfectly matched ours with a girl, girl, boy, and girl. Lastly, in September came Nella Lu who was the third child and third daughter of Alex and Jason. It was sweet that the parents of both Lucy and Nella Lu incorporated Luana's name into their child's name. So, now the total was 14 grandchildren. Our quiver was certainly overflowing. This would remind me of the song by Matt Redman, titled <u>Blessed Be the Name</u>, in which the line goes "You give and take away, but my heart will choose to say, blessed be the name of the Lord."

This also was the year that Luana and I turned 60 – her in May and me in July. I wrote a post to honor her so I thought I would share it here.

Today my sweet Luana is 60 years old. I obviously expected that it would look differently than it does, but we do not have the luxury to dictate how our lives will unfold. I want to take this time to honor her in the way she deserves on this very special day.

When Lou Gehrig made his famous farewell speech at Yankee Stadium, knowing he was dying with ALS, he said that he was the luckiest man alive. Well, I feel the same way in that having the privilege of being married to Luana for the past 38 years, I am the luckiest man alive. Yes, walking down this road of Alzheimer's has been extremely difficult, but I can honestly say that if I had known it would happen, I would have still married her anyway. The richness of the first 31 years dwarfs the pain of the past seven.

This past weekend with all of the kids in town, we had a birthday dinner for Luana (at Chuy's - our kid's favorite). As we usually do for birthdays, we all went around and said what we like about that person or a favorite memory. Some of the things said are very illustrative of who she is. One said that Luana acts as much like Jesus as any other person on earth that I have known. Having lived with her, I can say that I agree and that that is just naturally who she is. She is the same at home as she is with anyone she meets. She does not have to put on her "Christian" face as it is always on. Another person said that she is like a mirror into my soul when I am around her. I watch her and how she acts around other people and am convicted of my own sin without her ever having to say a word. One last thing, is that she is one of very few people who is just as comfortable around the president of a company as she is around a homeless person. She is not intimidated by either and treats them both the same. I could go on and on about her accolades, and many times we tend to focus on a person's good traits, neglecting the bad, but with Luana these comments are not exaggerations.

The man I am now has a lot to do with the grace and mercy of God and the power of the Holy Spirit to change lives, but it also has a lot to do with Luana. In our early days of marriage, I was self-centered, focused on school and my career and away from the home a lot. Being around someone like Luana has a tendency to rub off on you, and that is exactly what happened. She did not preach to me, call me out, or play games. She just continued to be who she is, and loved me and was very patient with me, praying for me the whole time. She was always supportive of me and was my best cheerleader, working to put me through school and then encouraging me that I was the "best" doctor. She gave me the freedom to pursue all that God had for me and did not resent any of it. She is truly a selfless person.

So, on this very special day for her I just want to say thanks for all you have done and for who you are. There are many lives who have been changed and impacted by your life. I love you.

As I said before, the curse for Alzheimer's is fairly flat for several years (and hers was for 5-6 years) but then it goes downhill pretty quickly after that. The years of 2014 – 2015 saw a huge decline in her functional abilities in so many areas:

I had always thought it interesting that when I would do a MMSE (mini mental status exam) on a patient, there was the question involving a simple 3 step command. It seemed so easy as to be silly. It was to 1) fold the paper in half 2) put it on the floor 3) raise the right hand. But as I have lived with an Alzheimer's spouse, I totally see the rationale for this question in the exam. Over the past few years, it has gotten more and more difficult for Luana to do even the simple tasks that I ask her to do. At first, it seemed like it was just that she would forget what I had said. But more and more it was obvious that she could not follow the command. Certainly, the most difficult tasks for her are multistep commands. It might be something like asking her to go upstairs and get me a drink in a cup with ice. Invariably, she would come down with something different. So now, I am very careful to only ask her to do simple one step commands.

I really wonder what must go through her mind when confronted with a command. At times it is almost comical in that she would often do the exact opposite of what I was asking her to do. The problem is that she is always wanting to help me and I want to try and honor that as much as I can. Unfortunately, it is most always easier to do things by myself, but that is not the best thing to do. What I really have to deal with is getting frustrated with her when she cannot understand what I am trying to say. I know in my mind that it is not her fault but, in the moment, it is so hard to understand why she cannot do it. One of the big things I am praying for is the grace to have patience with her during these times.

So how do I work with her to accomplish tasks? The first thing is to keep the command simple, not only as a single vs multistep command but also one that is straightforward and easy to understand. The next thing is to model what you want her to do by hands on. Then often you have to repeat the command over and over again. Remember as well, that it is just as frustrating for her as she wants to do the right thing.

This next one has to do with dressing, which as I mentioned earlier is one of the five major ADLs, and now she was starting to lose those. We grade the loss of ADLs on a scale of 1 to 4, with 1 being no help needed, 2 requiring stand by assistance, 3 indicating moderate help needed and 4 being full help.

But as I navigate this disease with my sweet wife, I find that the ADLs are far more complex than just "some assistance required". Let's take the task of dressing. What is actually required to accomplish this seemingly simple activity? One has to pick out clothes that are appropriate (weather and covering), and hopefully match. Then, he/she has to be able to put them on in the proper order (underwear before pants and top before a sweater). And lastly, one must be able to button, snap, buckle or whatever to finish the process. As the disease progresses, a person may require help in any of these steps, or eventually, all of them. But what I have found are some more interesting quirks to this process that I thought I would share. I am not sure if this applies across the board but I would not be surprised.

Luana has never been a flashy or trendy dresser, but has always dressed in the current style, with good taste in what goes together and what looks good on her. So much has changed that I will just have to describe it to you. The first thing is that she tends to wear the same thing over and over again now, sometimes two or more days in a row, if I do not stop her. A side note is that she does get mad at me if I point out that she wore something just yesterday and should not wear it today. I think there are a couple of reasons for this. The first of course, is that she does not remember what she wore yesterday, and if she liked it then, there is a good likelihood she will like it today as well. But another reason is that she does not put her clothes up in the closet or the drawers. I try to do it, but it is hard to keep up with, and she gets mad if I say anything or do it in front of her. So, she will see something laying out and just pick it up to wear again. Also, she will just pick the first thing in her drawer rather than looking all through it, and when I do put her clothes back in the drawer they are usually on top. I guess I could be proactive and put them on the bottom instead.

The other thing is that she does not always wear what is appropriate for the occasion. At this point, I have to step in, and of course I get a lot of grief there. I am more than happy to pick out her clothes, but she still knows enough to know that she does not want that. I guess somewhere in her memory is the fact that I have never been the best dresser or had the best tastes in clothes. My siblings got those genes, but not me.

And lastly, is the area of finishing the product. She has a lot of different jewelry, but only wears the same thing every day. She rarely puts on any make up now unless her sister helps her. Fortunately, she still looks pretty darn good for almost 60 and I really don't care about it, so it does not bother me. But it is totally different from in the past. She is still good about taking baths, but I am not in there so I am not sure how well she really cleans herself. So, in the ADL box, I would have to check that she can dress, but there is so much more to it than that.

As we have seen, Luana's writing skills deteriorated to the point where she was no longer able to continue to write her journal. But there is so much more to cognition, and that is the conundrum that is Alzheimer's. Most people think that it is just about recent memory, and certainly that it is the most obvious characteristic of the disease (actually the true name for this is episodic declarative memory). But to be true Alzheimer's, one has to have defects in multiple areas of cognition. This post gives a little insight into Luana's defects at this time.

Reading, Riting, and Rithmatic

These three Rs have been the foundation for learning for thousands of years. It has been fun as my grandchildren grow up, to be able to follow with them through this learning process and see them progress. As a parent one does not always appreciate it, since you are busy rearing them and see them daily so the increments are so small. But for grandparents, the increments are larger and we have the time to stop and wonder.

For Alzheimer's patients, the process is in reverse. And as exciting as it is to watch kids learn and develop, it is equally excruciating to watch your spouse lose the ability to do those things. For Luana, the first thing to go was mathematics. I think the first thing I noticed was her inability to manage the checkbook. Remember what that is? I may be dating myself, but in the not-too-distant past, we paid for things with checks and had little booklets where we recorded the expenses and then subtracted that from the total to see how much was left in the account. At the end of each month, I would look through the booklet and "balance" the checkbook. There got to be so many mistakes in putting down the correct amount of the expense, and then also in the subtracting, that I finally had to take that job away from her. We then went to putting all of the expenses on Quicken, but she had trouble doing that as well. She would try to do Sudoku early on in the course of the disease and at first, she could do the simplest level but has not been able to do it at all for a number of years.

She has trouble doing simple calculations such as figuring out a tip amount, so when she goes out to eat her friends have to put in that amount for her. Nor is she able to figure out change when spending cash. Not specifically math, but in a similar vein is the inability to read a non-digital clock. Nor can she figure out minutes or hours until the next event. Along the same line, is not being able to determine the number of days until an important event. We don't really stop and think how much we use math in our daily lives.

The next thing to go was her writing. She used to journal her prayers every morning but as the disease progressed, she had more and more difficulty writing down her thoughts. This would involve misspelling of simple words that she has always known. Then also she would have trouble formulating a complete sentence that makes sense. And then it got to the point where she could not remember how to write certain letters. Two things really stand out to me that exemplify this. One was last year when I redid my will and we met with the attorneys to sign the originals. She could write her first name, but could not for the life of her, write a G for her middle initial. Even when I wrote it out for her to copy, she could not do that. The second thing was when I had gotten a card for her to write a short note before mailing it. She could not even write a line that was comprehensible. Those kinds of things break my heart, as they show so vividly her mind slipping away.

And then there is reading. She has never been a fast reader, but over the years it has gotten slower and slower to the point where she could not finish a book at all. Part of that, of course, is that she forgets what she read, so it is not as interesting to her. One time when we were on a trip, she brought a book and she read the first chapter 15 times, not realizing that she had already read it. But lately, I have noted problems in knowing words and meanings. At night we will do a devotional book and I will have her read, and it is painful watching her try to pronounce the words and continually lose her place on the page and not understand what the words mean. Unfortunately, she sees this and realizes that she is having trouble, which makes it even more agonizing to me. But as always, she is not deterred and wants to keep trying. I admire that so much in her. It makes me love her all the more.

And lastly in this chapter, I will talk about another routine task that she could no longer do and that I had to take over. And like cooking, it was not one that I wanted to have to do. But it is part of the role of the caregiver, and you do what you have to do to keep the ship moving.

There are many activities that we all do as a part of our daily lives that virtually no one really enjoys doing, but are a necessary activity. Two of those are washing clothes and ironing. For us, this has been the last bastion of household work that Luana has been able to do. But alas, that wall is coming down as well. In these things, there is no clear event that signals it is over, but an accumulation of mistakes that, over a period of time, lets you know that it is time. Again, it is something that you, as the spouse, do not just come home one day and say your washing days are over. That is, unless you really want to get a shower of tears. What I have discovered (mostly through the hard way) over the years as the best way to do this, is to first offer my help in doing the activity and then we see it as a shared activity. Then, over time, I take over more and more of it, allowing her to do what she can. Fortunately, she has been pretty easy with this approach and eventually allows me to take over completely. Maybe she is smart, like Tom Sawyer and Huck Finn, and just making me think I am taking over because she cannot, when in reality, she didn't want to do it in the first place. But I digress.

The ironing was the first to go and has been going on for a long time. This is something that she, unlike most people in the world, actually liked to do. But I started to notice that my shirts were put into my closet with the collars all bent out of shape. Then one got ruined with a hole burnt into it. I also started to worry about the iron being left on all day with it being a fire hazard. The problem with ironing is that it is the one activity that I never have learned how to do. And I really have no desire to learn. So, it was not something I could take over. Instead, I started to get the shirts out of the dryer while still hot and hang them up right away. Most of mine are easy wear, so it works out pretty well. I also wear a lab coat over my shirt at work, so who cares if it is a little wrinkled? I know my mother would, but she is gone.

The washing has been more recent and gradual. I first noticed that a few of my clothes came back with white patches on them. It seems that she was using Clorox for some reason and just pouring it in directly. So, I just removed the Clorox from the laundry room. Next, I noticed that some clothes were coming out of the washer with cakes of detergent on them. I watched one day and she was just putting way too much detergent in the wash. Then, I started observing her more and more, and found she was putting all types of clothes together, washing sensitive clothes in hot water and washing a load most every day (we really can do it once a week). I also noticed she never cleaned the lint trap, so I had to be diligent to do it regularly. With all of this, I knew it was time to step in and take it over. So, that now puts all of the household chores on me. I am not complaining, as I am able to do it and as long as I am organized, I can fit it all in. It just leaves less time for doing other things. But as they say "that is life".

Chapter Eighteen

Caregiving

2015

As a physician, I have seen hundreds, if not thousands of patients with Alzheimer's and other dementias, and thus I knew a lot about it and I knew a lot of the disabilities they exhibited and have counseled countless numbers of caregivers. But I was surprised by how much of the day-to-day life of the patient and caregiver that I did not know. As her condition deteriorated throughout 2014 and 2015, I received a baptism of new understandings and insights into this disease. Part of that was the impetus for my blog. It also gave me new ammunition with which to give my patients and their caregivers.

I am going to go through a lot of issues that I had not known about, but which are important when caring for a demented patient. But first, I have to give a quote from my granddaughter, Molly, who was five at the time, which is precious. She and Luana had been particularly close and she just loved when Luana was visiting her. One day, she told her mother that she was missing Mimi and she was sad. It just turned out that they were coming to Waco for some event and they drove by the house to see us for a short visit.

This is a quote from her mother, Amy: "Lastly, I wanted to share something Molly said last year. She was really missing my mom and we ended up going to Waco anyway, so we got to see her. After we left, I said, 'Molly, did it do your heart good to be with Mimi?' and she replied, 'That's what it always does.' Anyone who knows my mom agrees that being around her does your heart good. She is one of a kind and I am so thankful God made her my mother."

Now here is a montage of the new things I was learning:

> Last weekend Luana and I went to the lake house. I spent the morning mowing the grass, weed eating and trimming trees. We had to get back so we left around 2:00 and planned to eat some lunch in Corsicana. Luana was hungry and as we approached, I told her to think about where she wanted to eat. After about 5 minutes she could not come up with a single idea of a place or type of food to eat. This is in a town we have driven through and stopped for lunch or dinner over 100 times and know pretty much every restaurant there. I started thinking about this, and realized that she no longer has the capacity to conceptualize things in her mind and bring that to her conscious mind. It is something we do automatically and without thinking. We pull from our memories those things that we need, and use them to make decisions. People with Alzheimer's do not have that ability. I think part of it is that those memories are not there to pull from. But I think there is another aspect to it as well. I cannot really put it into words as well as I would like, but I think they just lose the ability to think abstractly. If it is not there, it does not exist.

This is what I call conceptualization. I am not sure it is a real word but it sounds good and fits the situation.

There are numerous areas where this plays out, so it is not just a theoretical idea. One thing is getting dressed in the morning. She cannot conceptualize what she has in the closet, so she has to go and look at each item. But then, she also cannot conceptualize what the items will look like together, so there are some interesting combinations. Another thing is in decorating. Luana has always been good at making our house look beautiful and stylish, but now that has all changed. Thinking about it, I see that it is the same problem of not being able to conceptualize what looks good without it actually being there. The more I explore this concept, the more I realize it explains a lot of the disabilities of Alzheimer's patients. And in many ways, it is like a young child who does not have the memories to draw from to be able to conceptualize, and therefore is very concrete in his thinking. So, also Alzheimer's patients tend to become more like kids as the disease progresses.

And then there is this thought about love.

"...for better or for worse, for richer or for poorer, in sickness and in health..." go the words spoken every weekend of the year. I would venture to say that most couples getting married do not even think what those words mean. They have a lot of other things on their minds; especially the guys. Even well into the first year of marriage, those thoughts rarely come into view. And unfortunately, down the road when they do, most couples ditch it for the supposed greener grass on the other side of the fence. For those of us taking care of spouses with Alzheimer's, those words hit home every day and it is a strain to keep reminding yourself of your commitment.

This post is entitled love, not necessarily the romantic type, but what the Bible calls agape love. The English language is very poor at describing love. We "love" everything from football to Dr Pepper to our wives – and I hope those are not all equal. The Greeks were much better, using four different words to express those feelings. I will not go into all of their meanings but want to focus on the highest form of love – agape. It is the word used in many weddings, recited from I Corinthians 13. But though it is used in this context, it really has nothing to do with romantic love and is used to describe the love of God for man and between two individuals. It is also the word used in the most familiar passage in the Bible, John 3:16, describing how much God loved the world (that means us).

So, what is this love? It is a self-sacrificial type of love, giving of itself freely and demanding nothing in return. It places value on another person, not because of what they have done, but simply because it chooses to do so. It is not a feeling and something you fall in and out of, but it is a deliberate choice. Does that sound like something Hollywood has in mind in its movies?

Finally, what does this have to do with a blog on Alzheimer's? Everything really! You tend to lose romantic love when your spouse does not even know who you are (we are not quite there yet). So, what holds a couple together through these difficult months and years? It is this agape love. It is the realization that you made a commitment to another person for life, and knowing that she would do the same for you if the roles were reversed. It is a love that seeks nothing in return – for in reality you do get very little back. But don't get me wrong. By this I do not mean a white knuckled holding on or an "I'm stuck" type of love. That is just enduring a bad situation because you know you should. I am speaking of real love – the kind of love that should be written about, but does not make for good movies. It is a love that says I am thankful to serve you in this way because of all of the wonderful years you have given to me.

I am thankful to God that He has given to me this type of love for Luana. I cannot explain it nor can I pull it up on my own. It is a God given love. It is there when I can look into her face and gaze into her eyes and see the old Luana, and am drawn to her. It is there when she asks me the same thing for the tenth time and I do not get angry. It is there when I am cooking dinner after coming home from work and resent it, but I press on anyway. It is there when I need to get some work done at home, but I stop and go on a walk with her because that is what she wants to do. I can honestly say that right now I would rather be with Luana in her condition, than with any other woman. I do not say that because I am good – I say it because God is good, and He works His goodness in us.

But caregiving is not always pure and we don't always show that kind of love and patience. In fact, there are numerous times where we blow it and mess up. I certainly did – and still do.

As I stood there watching her cry and walk away, I asked myself how I could have let it happen again. The bottom line is that I blew it again. By blew it, I mean that I had lost my patience and had raised my voice to her. She is very sensitive to that and it makes her cry. Then, I feel terrible because I know it is not her fault and I want so much to treat her well. I resolve in my mind that it will not happen again, but I know deep down that it will. Because there is no way that it cannot. I am human and this struggle against this devastating disease does not end quickly or easily. It takes no prisoners. So, sooner or later my patience will once again come to an end, and I will raise my voice to her and she will cry. I will again feel bad and the cycle will go on and on. The only good thing about Alzheimer's is that her memory is short and she does not remember my making her cry. An hour later she is hugging me and thanking me for taking such good care of her. But I don't forget. The memory of the sad look in her eyes is enough to make me not want to ever do it again. And while her forgiveness is real, if only because it is forgotten, I have a much more difficult time forgiving myself.

As I have been thinking about this, I had a startling revelation. This is exactly how it is with us in our relationship with God. We sin and it hurts Him (at least I imagine it does) and we feel terrible about it. We resolve that we will never do it again, and we try very hard not to, but alas we find ourselves right back at it. This is the struggle that the apostle Paul describes in Romans 7. He finally asks who will save him from this body of death. Of course, the answer is Christ. We cannot stop sinning on our own, but through the power of the Holy Spirit, we can overcome. One difference for us with God is that we cannot really look directly into His eyes and see the hurt that is in them. I think that if we could, we would sin a lot less. But He also offers forgiveness readily, and in the same way we have a much harder time forgiving ourselves.

In the end, it is important to realize that I do not have to be perfect in my caring for Luana. None of us are and we will continue to make mistakes, no matter how hard we try. Even if I were perfect, that would not be an encouraging word to the millions of caregivers around the world. What everyone wants to hear is that the pain, the loneliness, the sacrifices and yes, even the mistakes are all worth it. And on that account, I say a resounding yes.

We tend to focus too much on what the loved one can't do or how badly we mess up, but in the end, we need to focus more on the positive.

The other day my daughter texted me a comment that really stuck with me. She said "One of my favorite parts of having mom here is waking up to hearing on the monitor all of the kids in bed with her, giggling and talking for the longest time. They all go in there right when they wake up." It really struck a chord with me and made me so happy. I am always having to deal with all she cannot do, so it is so good to hear what she really can do in a positive way. And what is so nice about kids is they do not care how much you can remember, or even so much what you bought them for their birthday. What they care about is you being there and giving them undivided attention. No one does that better than Mimi. Even the oldest girl knows that something is wrong with Mimi and that she cannot do all the things that other grandmothers do, but it does not bother her in the least. She still loves to go in the bed with her and talk and play. We can all learn a lot from that.

One of the things I like that Luana's sister does, is to always remind me of the times when Luana acts like Jesus. It varies but is usually a comment she makes or something she does involving someone who is less fortunate. Even though she cannot discuss doctrine, Luana can still be sensitive to the work of the Holy Spirit inside of her. It is often very humbling to those of us around her. Many times, someone will give us news of a friend who is sick or in need and we may all be discussing it, when out of the blue Luana will say "Let's just pray about that right now."

It is interesting, because Luana is one who always focused on the positive in all situations and especially with people. So, it comes full circle as we try to focus on the positive in her. And it certainly applies to all caregivers dealing with Alzheimer's patients. It helps in so many different ways. It helps the patient by putting them in situations where they have a much better chance of succeeding. It helps the caregiver by giving them something to aim toward in a positive way. But it also helps the caregiver by reminding us that the patient really is a human being and still has value.

And then there is this:

For those of us who care for an Alzheimer's patient, milestones carry a different and more ominous meaning. The milestones I am talking about are negative ones, marking points of further decline. This past week, I was able to see two new milestones in the life of my sweet wife. The first was eating dinner of pork tenderloin that our wonderful neighbors had made for us. Luana could not figure out how to use the knife and fork to be able to cut the pork, so for the first time, I had to cut it for her. Shortly after that, I was trying to tell her how to get something out of the cabinet and told her to open the one on the right. She opened left and I corrected her and said right. She gave me a confused look so I asked her if she knew what was right and left and she said no. I had suspected it for some time, but had never actually asked her. It was very sobering, as it was a definite milestone marking further decline in her level of functioning.

But for me, it was a silent marker. I did not post a picture on Instagram and I made no note on Facebook. It was not something I wanted to call my children and tell them about. That is the thing about Alzheimer's – there is a lot of silent suffering. Most all caregivers would agree with me in this regard. Again, I am not mentioning this to elicit sympathy but just to make known what is. Each mile marker is a reminder that this disease is a progressive degenerative disorder, and it is going to continue to go downhill. A lot of the time you go throughout your day thinking that this is the way it is and you have adjusted to it, but then there are these times that you are reminded that that is not the way it is going to be. It is going to get harder.

Chapter Nineteen

Full Time Care

2016

Once again, the calendar turned and we were now in 2016 and with it, life was about to get even harder. I had already given up the Bible study I was doing at the Manna House, which was the last activity that I had held onto, so that I could focus entirely on Luana. I was still teaching my class at Baylor and playing tennis one afternoon a week, but nothing else.

Shortly into the new year, another of the major crises occurred. During most of the days while I was at work, Luana was with her sister. Cathy was getting busier as she adjusted to life in Waco, and had a part time job with Weight Watchers and was getting more and more meetings with that. Often, she would bring Luana to the meetings, but that was getting harder to do. It was becoming more and more of a burden on her. I had told her and her husband repeatedly that I was appreciative of all that she did, but that none of it was expected and she could back off of any or all at any time.

At the same time, it was becoming obvious that it was not safe for Luana to be home by herself at all. This was a conversation that I was going to have to have with her. I was not looking forward to it. Sure enough, it did not go down well. I sat down and tried to explain that Cathy was not able to watch her as much as she had, and that because of the progression of the disease, she was not safe alone. I told her that we would need to get someone in the house to sit with her. She just burst into tears and could not understand at all why she could not be by herself. She told me that she had not done anything wrong (which she had not) or caused any problems (again, not yet). But I was firm in my decision, and determined to keep her safe. Many times, I have sat across from caregivers and told them that they needed to have the difficult conversation with their loved one. I was not going to back out of this. It hurt so much to watch her cry like that, and even now as I write this I am welling up with tears. I did not want to have to have someone stay with her. I did not want her condition to deteriorate so much. I did not want for her to have this disease at all. But it did not matter what I wanted. It is what it is.

Fortunately, Luana is pretty passive and after a while she settled down and accepted her fate. Not all patients do this, and many have kicked out paid caregivers, not letting them into their homes. I have recommended several agencies to patients and caregivers over the years, so I knew what to do. I called Visiting Angels (I knew the owner of the local franchise) and they came out to evaluate the situation and we settled on the hours. Cathy was still with her several days so she tag teamed with them.

This situation severely limited my activities as well. I had to be home until the caregiver arrived in the morning and I had to leave work to make it home by 5:30. One of the few nice things about electronic records is that I could finish up and do my "paper work" on my computer at home. But I could no longer meet a friend for breakfast or for a dinner. If I wanted to go to get something at Home Depot (which I often did), I would have to take Luana with me. When I would go to the gym to work out (I had had to give up running due to my knees), I had to bring Luana with me and have her sit in the lobby while I did my work out. And of course, on the weekends we were together 24/7.

And together we were. By this point she did not like to be left alone, even in another part of the house. She wanted to be right with me, wherever I was. I had heard this from patients and I was not surprised, but it can get oppressive at times. We all need our space. When I was at my desk doing work, she would sit in a chair right beside me. If I was out working in the shop then she would come out there. If I was in the garden, then I would bring a chair for her while I worked. Then she was not satisfied with just being with me, but wanted to "help". This was always worse than me doing it by myself, because she could never understand what I was telling her to do, and would invariably do it wrong and I would have to do it all over. I understood her desires, and I wanted to allow her to help, but it was very difficult – and I lost it a few times.

We did take some trips that year as well. We went on a quick trip out to southern California to my niece's wedding. We went a little early and got to explore a little of the area. It really is beautiful and we drove along Highway 1 which hugs the coast and gives you a pretty vista around almost every curve. Or, if you get tired of the ocean, you can look the other way up into the mountains. Then, in May we went back to Michigan where I again combined a visit to my kids with a CME course. It is beautiful up there that time of year as well. But travelling, especially by plane, with an Alzheimer's patient is stressful, even if everything goes well. Going through security is the worst, as I have to explain to the TSA agent that she has Alzheimer's and cannot follow the directions that they require. They then have to call and get a lady to come and walk her through, and do a pat down. I have to carry all of her stuff and do everything, while always watching out so that she does not get lost. Fortunately, she is not a wanderer, so she doesn't just walk away, but she cannot follow well. What I mean by this is that if I am walking, and get ahead of her (which I typically do as she is much slower these days), she will frequently either stop or walk in a different direction. She just does not pay attention. I have lost her many times this way (once outside the Baylor football stadium with thousands of people milling around – luckily some friends of ours noticed her and kept her with them until I made it back), so now I have to walk slower and keep looking around to make sure she is there. Then there is always the restroom problem. I am an old man now, and I have to go more than she does. Since she does not wander, I can instruct her to stand right outside while I go in. But it is hard when she has to go. One of the nice things about airports is that they have family bathrooms, so this works out well and I can take her in there and help her. There are just so many little things that most people would never think about.

In June, we drove to Winter Park, CO and rented a large 6-bedroom house near the slopes and all of us met there (24 of us at this time) and stayed in that one house. It was kind of wild as you can imagine, but it was a lot of fun. Those trips are nice since there are so many people around who know her and are able and willing to help out. The drive was long but we did not have to deal with the airport thing. Luana was still able to enjoy being around the little ones, but was interacting less and less which was so sad to see. For her to enjoy and play with them was one of the few things that tempered the anguish of this disease. And I had always felt that it was God's blessing in the midst of the suffering that we had so many of them. But even that small bit of joy was also eventually taken away.

Then, I did one more trip – this my annual college football trip with my brother-in-law – this year to Knoxville, TN to see the Tennessee Volunteers. It, like Baylor, is one of three stadiums right on a river. As usual, we went early and did some hiking in the Smoky Mountains and it was great. I am thankful that my daughters were able to tag-team and watch Luana while we went. They are always so willing to help, even though they all have young children and lead busy lives. This is not the case for every Alzheimer's patient. I take advantage of this because I know that I need it, and it has the added benefit of them getting to take care of her by themselves, and see how difficult it is. You can know it intellectually, but you really don't know it until you do it for a few days.

How was I doing in all of this? I'm not going to lie to you – it was hard. It was just constant with no relief – a daily grind is the best way I can describe it. And I had it better than most, because I was younger and still working, and was able to get away during the day on Monday through Friday. On the other hand, you could say it was worse, in that I had to work all day and then come home and work all night. Luana was clearly on the steep downward part of the curve and getting worse rapidly. It seemed like there was something new that she could no longer do almost every week. It was hard to find a rhythm. Somewhere around this time, I made the decision to take her off of her Alzheimer's meds, as they were clearly no longer working (if indeed they ever did anything to begin with). This is a personal decision between the caregiver and their physician, and many never want to stop, hoping that they do something. I could not discern any difference off of the meds.

There were times when I was not sure that I could keep going. I was having to do more and more – already I was doing everything related to the home – of Luana's personal care, and many were things I never thought that I would be having to do. I will discuss many of those things later. Add to that, the reality that you get virtually no reward for what you do. Earlier on, she would tell me thanks when I would do something for her, and it was helpful that she knew I was doing what she could no longer do. But at this point, there was none of that – no positive reinforcement. But, at each stage God gave me the grace to do what I needed to do, and to do it with a positive attitude, and He gave me the strength to keep going. One of the defense mechanisms you use to get through this, is detachment. The reason for this, is that if you thought about all of the loss on a daily basis, you would just be spent emotionally, and be crying continuously. I wrote a post on this at about this time.

> Today I was having lunch with my brother and we were discussing Luana and the emotional toll it exacts on the caregiver and the rest of the family. He mentioned a term I had never heard which he had gotten from another program – detachment with love. As he said it, the term instantly resonated with me. I had been explaining to him that as a physician, I often had to detach myself from my patients emotionally, in order to care for them properly. This is not to say that I didn't care – just the opposite – I cared too much for I have cared for many of my patients for over 20 -25 years. When they get sick, you have to show some emotion, because there is no way not to. We are not machines. But if you let yourself go, the emotions would be overwhelming, since it is repeated multiple times over many patients. Therefore, we have to detach a little and compartmentalize the disease from the person, so as to be able to continue to care for them in an effective way.

> The conversation moved from that to my attitudes toward Luana. I discussed that I had taken a similar approach with her, not necessarily consciously, but realistically. I still love her without reservation, but I have detached somewhat emotionally. This is a defense mechanism, and is necessary because

otherwise one's emotional energy would be spent early on. So, what does that exactly look like? It does not mean that I do not care – it is necessary because I care too much. I am sad when she gets frustrated or when she cries. It breaks my heart when there is one more new thing that she cannot do. I tear up when I see our friends do things with their grandchildren that Luana can never do. But those emotions stop there. I do not let my mind dwell on those things, and I do not let myself wonder about the future and what it will hold. Occasionally, I will forget and find myself dwelling on something she can no longer do, and I just begin to sob uncontrollably. I think from time to time even that is healthy, just not too often. And not where she can see.

But detachment without love would be akin to abandonment. Love is the tether that holds it all together. That would be to treat her with tenderness and compassion. It would be responding with patience when she asks you the same thing ten times. That would be to put your arm around her and tell her you still love her, and that she is stuck with you. It would be helping her get dressed in the morning, brush her teeth at night, cut up her meat or tie her shoes. Love is still spoken, but even more so, it is lived out each day in the daily things of life with her. One of my greatest pleasures now is when

I hear her say "I appreciate the way you love me". That is when I know I am doing it right. Thank you, Lord, for those moments and the grace to do it.

The other thing that helps is to keep it all in perspective. It is so easy to think that you are the only one who is struggling, and having to go through all of this suffering. You get focused on self. But this year I had a friend who was dying with ALS, and another whose wife was dying with metastatic breast cancer. That helps you keep your attitude better. Very few people get through this world without suffering.

Chapter Twenty

A Little Help From Our Friends

2017

ThatBy the time 2017 rolled around, Luana was well into the steep downhill part of the curve. Every month it seemed like there was something new that Luana could not do. It is the opposite of a little child where every month they seem to be doing a new thing – and we all rejoice in that new thing they can now do. But with Alzheimer's, it is heartbreaking, not to mention more work for the caregiver.

We have already seen some of the big things that she was no longer able to do – cooking, finances, driving, laundry. But over this year or so, there were multiple smaller things which I had to do for her, many of which I never thought I would be doing. We can just follow a typical day and see all of the things that come up.

About this time, she was becoming incontinent – first of urine and then later of stool as well. But early on, she was still mostly continent, and first thing in the morning I would put her on the toilet and she would have a bowel movement. That was good though I would have to wipe her bottom. That is tough on both the caregiver and the patient (though by this time Lu had lost all sense of modesty). It really is one of those things you never expect to do when you say "I do". She was not able to dress herself, so I picked out her clothes and helped her get dressed. It is a scary thought for me to be picking out clothes, as I have never been accused of having good taste. But I think I actually did pretty well. I even had to pick out and buy her new clothes, and I do say that I learned what looked good on her (even my kids thought I was doing pretty well). One little side note is the problem of trying on clothes at the store, if the dressing rooms are for women only, because Luana could not do it herself.

For a while, I even put a little make up on her. I had no idea what I was doing, but my daughter taught me what to do. It was not much but just a soft touch. Next, we would make it to the kitchen for breakfast. We did not do anything fancy – mostly just cereal – and I would get it ready and then I would have to feed her every bite. After cleaning up, I was ready for the sitter to come, but first I had to brush her teeth. Again, something you never think about doing for/to your spouse, and it is a lot harder than you think, especially when they cannot follow your commands. After work, I would get home and prepare dinner and then sit down and feed her. I didn't bathe her every night, but usually 3-4 times a week. At first, she was able to get into the tub and when I realized that she was not actually bathing herself, I took on that role. Another small thing that I would do once a week while in the tub, was to shave her legs. I never thought that I would be doing that. After a while, it got harder and harder to get her out of the tub, so I started giving her a shower. That is difficult to do and stay dry, so I would just get in with her and we would do it together.

I would then get her dressed in her pajamas and put her to bed. Eventually, over the course of the year, she deteriorated to the point where she was totally incontinent. She was frequently wetting her underwear, and of course her clothes which meant more laundry. Often, it was the bedsheets as well, so we had to go to diapers – first just at night and then all the time. Changing wet diapers is not difficult, but changing dirty ones is a huge challenge. For me, I found that the best way was to have her stand by the toilet and I would cut off the diaper and then use toilet paper/wipes to clean her. There were times when I would have to bite my lip and not say anything. I knew it wasn't her fault, but it is a most unpleasant thing to have to do (much worse than cleaning a dirty diaper of a baby), and at times you are tired and you just want to scream.

I go through all of this for two reasons. One is just to show how far and how fast she went down during this period of time. The second and most important, is to show the depth of God's grace. If you had told me early on that I would be doing all of these things, I would have run fast the other way. But amazingly, God gave me the grace for each new step along the way. I was able to do it and to do it (most of the time) with a loving heart and to treat her well, as she deserved. It certainly was not in my power to do that.

The other thing that happened during this period, is how neighbors stepped up in a big way. When I had my heart bypass surgery back in 2009, the Lord taught me a big lesson. I was helpless and needed lots of help. I could not do it on my own. I had always been the one to help people, but I never liked to ask for help. One day as I was praying, I felt like the Lord reminded me of a truth. That truth was that I got a huge blessing by helping other people. He then spoke to my spirit, "Are you going to deprive other people of a blessing that they would get by helping you, simply by being stubborn and prideful and not asking for help?" That hit me like a ton of bricks, but it was the best thing that I learned from that trial. And I never realized how much it would help me down the road, when I would need lots of help with Luana. Now when people offer help, I say "Yes" and "Thank you".

Well, God sent many helpers my way. We have lived in the same house, in the same neighborhood for 35 years. It is a great neighborhood, and we are very blessed. One day, several years ago, a neighbor a few houses down the street offered to cook us a meal once a week. This offer was of her own free will, and I was blown away. I thought she would do this for a few weeks, and I was very thankful. But the meals kept coming for over two years, and only stopped when we put Luana in the memory care facility. You talk about faithful service. To make matters better, is that she is a very good cook. The problem I had was how to say thanks enough for such a sacrifice. I tried by giving her a gift card to our local grocery store from time to time, bringing some of the produce from my garden, and writing thank you notes every so often. But there is no way to repay that – and that is the point – you do not repay a gift – their reward is the blessing. Another neighbor down the street, who also is a great cook, has also brought meals on a consistent basis, and has had us over for dinner at her house many times. Even now, with Luana in the facility, she continues to bless me with food. Then, my neighbor across the street will text me occasionally that they have extra food that they have made, and want to know if I would like some. I have learned to even accept spontaneous surprises, which is hard for the planner in me.

But it is not just food either. Luana has three high school friends with whom she has stayed close all of these years. Over the past decade, we have gotten together with them and their husbands which is a lot of fun as we all get along very well. Two of them live in the DFW area and over the past several years, they would drive down once a month to spend the day with Luana. They continued to do this even after Luana went into the facility – that is until Covid hit. Luana loved these times and these friends were totally at ease with her in her demented state. One of them dealt with Alzheimer's in her mother for years, so she had a lot of experience. These friends really embody true selfless love.

Then there was the biggest surprise of them all. During this time, I had one of the students in my class tell me that she had been reading my blog and wanted to know if she could help out by sitting with Luana, so I could get some time away. This was out of the blue. I thought it would be best to have her meet Luana first, so we took her and her boyfriend out to eat. Immediately, I could see this was a good thing. She was so comfortable around Luana and she loved being with her. So, she stated coming one evening a week through the end of the semester. It was great for me in that I got some much-needed time by myself. But it was even better for Luana. She did not come over to sit with her and play on her cell phone the whole time. She had planned ahead and had different activities for them to do each night. This was when Luana could still walk and talk and do some things. I thought it would end with the semester, but she stayed in town over the summer and continued to come by each week through the summer and the whole next year – until she graduated and got married. Luana and I went to her wedding in Minnesota and had a great time. In addition to a special friendship with Kristen, I had the bonus of getting to know her fiancé (now husband) and we continued to connect and stay in touch even after they married and moved to Dallas. They are a precious couple. And to boot, he is a big sports and Baylor fan and we have lots of fun talking Baylor athletics.

Here was my blog about this at the time:

> Out of the blue one of my students in the spring class sent me an e mail. She had been reading this blog and had been stirred by the Holy Spirit to take action. (that in itself is a lesson for all of us). She tried to think of how she could help us, so she e-mailed me to see if she could come over one evening a week to sit with Luana, while I went out to run errands or whatever. I was shocked at the offer but I have learned over the past eight years to humble myself and allow people to help. When we let people help, it gives them a blessing, but when

we do not accept help, it deprives them of that blessing. So, I said sure, not really knowing if it would work out. Due to some scheduling conflicts, we did not connect until mid-July but eventually did. I thought it would be best first to take her out to dinner so Lu could meet her and it would not be awkward when she came to sit with her. We met and she and Lu hit it off immediately. The young Baylor student, Kristen, is incredibly sweet and just knew how to relate to Luana. She was respectful and not condescending. It reminded me a lot of the old Luana. That is a huge compliment.

Well, the next week she came and, except for a time when she was gone on vacation, she has been here each week. I thought it might end with the end of the summer but she has continued it on into the school year. What is so amazing is that she does not just come over and sit with her and watch TV. She is so creative with her. She will go through picture albums, go to the lake and watch the sun set, sing songs, walk along the dam. One day, she even went and got some water colors and they painted. Another day, she took her to an exotic animal store. Luana is so drawn to her. I have never seen her laugh so much as when she is with Kristen.

Chapter Twenty-One

Loneliness

2017

There was a lot going on during this time and I was having a hard time wrapping my brain around it all. One of the toughest things for me was the deterioration of her language functions. As I have said many times, Alzheimer's is a disease that involves multiple areas of cognition. Short-term memory is the most prominent in most people, and what we really associate with the disease, but it is by no means the only area. Language skills are also frequently lost. That can involve so many different functions – losing vocabulary, poor grammar, inability to write, concrete thinking, poor understanding, and later the ability to make complete sentences and eventually the ability to speak at all. I was not really prepared for this, as you can tell by the following blog post:

> "Can you pull that extension cord out of the plug for me?"
>
> "Okay"
>
> "But you are not doing it."

"What do you want?"

"The extension cord. The red one – right at the bottom of your feet."

"This one?"

"No, that is not an extension cord."

"Which one?"

"There is only one. It is right there in front of you. Ahhhhhhhhhhh. You are driving me crazy."

On and on it went that weekend. We were at our lake house on Cedar Creek Lake and I was finishing up a new deck we had built. Over and over, I asked her to get a tool for me and she could not do it, even when it was right there. It was like we were speaking two different languages, only a foreigner would at least be able to understand signs to get the object.

It was at that point that I really understood the value of words. Of course, I have always understood their value. I am an avid reader, and here I am writing this blog post every week. But, I really understood in the context of Alzheimer's disease, how crucial words are to convey meanings, ideas, tasks, feelings. There is so much here twirling around in my head on this subject. I hope I can put what I am thinking into words. Ha! There you have it. Words are by themselves important. A lot can be communicated just with single words. But then, so much more can be communicated when you put them into sentences. Remember when your children or grandchildren began to put words together? And then add inflection and tone and even body language, and so much more is opened up. Without trying to get too philosophical, words are what make us human. (Now I realize that there are certain individuals with disabilities who are not able to speak and they are just as much of a person, but I am speaking of the race in general). One more thought on words before I move on – even God in His creative power "spoke" the world into existence. And what does the apostle John use to describe Jesus? In the beginning was the Word. So yes, words are extremely important.

But back to Luana. As the disease has progressed, she has lost more and more the ability to use words in sentences, and even more so lately, to speak or understand words at all. It is so frustrating trying to have a conversation with her, as she will try to say something but she forgets the thought even before the end of the sentence. No amount of coaching or trying to drag it out of her will work. And then, when I ask her a question, it does not register with her at all. At dinner the other night, I was trying to initiate some conversation, so I asked her what her favorite color was. Her response was totally unrelated to what I had asked. But now, it is to the point where she does not understand specific words. If I asked her to point to something blue, she could not do it; nor could she name a color if I pointed to it. The idea of right and left is totally foreign to her. Even sign language is of no help. If I pointed up to show her something, she would just mimic me but not follow what I am trying to get her to see or do.

So, you can imagine how difficult life is on a day-to-day basis. We cannot sit and have conversation – it is frustrating even for the caretakers that come it to sit with her. At dinner we just sit and eat. There is no real communication, unless you count her asking how my day was ten times. She wants to help me in the tasks I am doing, but she cannot do so because she cannot follow what I am asking or need. Then, she gets frustrated and often will cry and I get very frustrated and will lose my cool. Yes, it does happen – far too often. Fortunately, and this is the only good thing about Alzheimer's, she quickly forgets and we are back on good terms. So, next time you speak to another person, think how critical and meaningful those words are and where you would be without them.

But, the ability to communicate verbally with Luana was not the only thing that was lost, and that also affected our relationship. This is where it is important to have a solid relationship to begin with, because Alzheimer's will stretch you and will reveal any cracks in the foundation like no other. Physical touch was another part of our lives that was lost.

> Physical touch is one of the most basic of human needs. But, we generally do not tend to see it that way. We know and understand hunger and thirst. These will not allow us to neglect them for long. But touch is one of those needs that does not have an immediate deprivation sensation. Numerous studies have shown that the lack of physical touch causes emotional scarring. Children growing up without touch have significant developmental abnormalities. On the other hand, touch can have a very positive effect in healing in those with a variety of illnesses. As a physician, I understand the value of touch, and use it daily in my practice. A good firm handshake, a pat on the shoulder, a good hug on my little old ladies goes a long way. In fact, I have had a few ladies get mad at me because they did not get a hug at the end of their appointment.

> So, what does this have to do with Alzheimer's? It is not something I had thought about a lot, nor is it anything I have discussed with my patients to any degree. But lately, I have come to realize how it is affecting me. Now I am not saying this is universal with Alzheimer's, and I may be more sensitive because I love hugs and physical touch. In fact, it is probably my number one love language. I am seeing that one of the things that some (if not most)

Alzheimer's patients lose, is the ability to do meaningful touch. By meaningful, I mean that the touch is not random – it has a purpose behind it. Certainly, these patients can physically touch others, but they have lost the ability to convey purpose in that touch.

Obviously, there are different kinds of touch in different situations. You touch patients differently from your brother or sister or your friend or your parent. And of course, you touch your spouse differently than all of the above. And that is what I am talking about now. I am not talking about sexual touch – that is a whole other topic for a whole other post (if I ever get the nerve). But I am speaking of that gentle but caressing touch that conveys to your partner that you love him and lets him know that he is still the one. It is that touch that says that I am still attracted to you. It may be a hug that lingers just a few seconds longer, or the gentle extra squeeze when holding hands. It could take the form of a back rub or a foot massage. I think you get the picture, and the list could go on and on, and for every person and every couple is different in how they express it. But, it is difficult to have a good marriage without it.

What got me thinking about this, is that I realized that it has been years since I have received that kind of touch. Luana is just not capable of that any longer. She still has love deep in her heart, but is not able to express it like she used to. Occasionally, in one of her more lucid moments, she will say that she is thankful for me caring for her. But that is the extent of it. So, where am I going with this idea other than to bemoan the loss? I think first it is important for caregiver spouses to realize this as another in a long list of things lost, and how it might affect you emotionally. Secondly, I think it is important for families and friends to be aware as well. Unfortunately, there is no healthy way to replace this loss. Spouses need to be careful to avoid getting into relationships in an attempt to meet that need. Sadly, I have seen patients who have cheated on their demented spouses. I do not advocate that at all. This is a topic that is rarely talked about, but is real and I wanted to bring it to light. I would appreciate comment from anyone who has experienced similar losses or have thoughts on the subject.

From here we have to go on and talk about a more difficult subject – the most intimate of all aspects of marriage – sexual intercourse. Read my post on this, and you will understand before I go on to the last in this series.

For a long time, I have wanted to write on this topic, but have been wary as I did not want to embarrass my children. I still do not want to embarrass them, but I think I can do it in a discreet way without any harm. I have written about general intimacy before, but never about physical intimacy – in a word – sex and the Alzheimer's patient. This is not something that is talked about a lot, nor written about for obvious reasons. But, it is an important topic, and I did not want to completely shy away from it.

At first thought, you may say gross, no way. But yes, it is something we have to deal with. I will say that even though I have taken care of hundreds, if not a thousand Alzheimer's patients, I do not have a lot of data on this from my patients. Presumably, they do not like to bring up the issue, or are too embarrassed. But, I do have some, and my own experiences as well, and I think I can extrapolate from them fairly accurately. Obviously, sexual practices vary widely even in the normal population, and with different age cohorts. That is no different in the Alzheimer's patients. But I do think I can make some pretty accurate generalizations.

First, is that in well over 90% of the couples with Alzheimer's, sexual encounters go down in frequency. There are many reasons for this, and I will try to outline as many as I can. One, is that most Alzheimer's patients are older, and usually the frequency has already diminished by then. Secondly, the caregiver is usually worn out by the end of the day, and is too tired to be interested in sex. (Much like the mothers of young children). Thirdly, Alzheimer's patients tend to be less interested in any kind of physical attraction, so even if the caregiver is interested, there is little response. Fourthly, and this may seem weird, but the patient seems to have forgotten "how" to engage in the act. Thus, even if they try, it is often not a positive experience. Then, there are other reasons such as no longer living at home or having someone in the house at all times to help care for them. There may be additional physical illnesses that inhibit the motivation or the ability.

Of course, there are exceptions and I know of some patients that go to the other extreme and are hypersexual. To be honest, that is almost always male Alzheimer's patients with female spouse caregivers. For these caregivers, it can be a very difficult road to navigate.

Despite these limitations, many caregivers are still interested in sexual activity. Early on in the disease, it is not as big a problem, but as the disease progresses, I would suggest going slowly and talking to your spouse, explaining what is going on so that they are not confused. You need to be sensitive and not force the issue if the spouse gets agitated or upset. You may have to limit your activities to lesser things, like kissing and hugging, but even these are often not as bipartisan as you might like.

I do want to add a word of extreme caution. Because the sexual (and for that matter the emotional) intimacy is not there, we need to be very careful not to look for or find it in other places. I am mostly talking to male caregivers, though it is not exclusively us. Too many times, I have seen my patient's spouse involved in immoral behavior. It is easy to turn to pornography or to start seeing another woman. Often, this can start out innocently by just spending time with a woman to have some real conversation. That leads to emotional intimacy, and often more. It can be very lonely, and it is not easy, but being faithful is worth it.

All of this – not being able to communicate, loss of touch, and loss of sexual intimacy – leads to the end result of loneliness on the part of the spouse caregiver. All of the major legs of a firm marital foundation have been removed. There is no way that it cannot happen. Here is a post I wrote on this a few years ago, but it is equally pertinent today.

There are so many things that I want to write about, that it is hard to pick one. Things come into my mind all throughout the day that I think would be helpful, but in the end, it is usually what is on my mind at the time that wins out. Tonight, it is loneliness. You might ask how you could be lonely when you live with someone all of the time, and it would be a good question. And I don't mean to make light of single men and women who really do walk into an empty house at the end of a day. That really is loneliness, and my heart goes out to them. Mine is a different kind, and I will try to explain.

I am very blessed in that I have lots of friends and family, and can call any of them at a moment's notice. I also have a job with a number of truly wonderful people with whom I can talk and share, and are a lot like family. I am engaged in a lot of activities that involve people – church, life group, teaching my class, sporting events, dinners, grandchildren, etc. So, I am not lonely because there are no people around my life. It is because of one particular person in my life.

There are lots of different types of relationships, but marriage is distinctly unique. There is a reason that marriage has survived intact for many millennia. There is a special bond of intimacy that is not matched in any other relationship. So many people say that their spouse truly is their best friend. Things happen during a day that you want to come home and share with your spouse. There may be a joyous event that you want to celebrate, and no one else would really appreciate it like a spouse. It could be hurt feelings that you could not share with anyone else. Then, there is so much history between the two of you such that just a look will bring a connection. I could go on and on, but those who have been married know what I am talking about.

With Alzheimer's patients, that is all gone. Certainly, it does not happen right away, but slowly but surely, the conversations get shorter and shorter. The sharing gets less and less. And the intimacy begins to fade away. Sure, there is a person there, but there is no relationship. She has lost her long-term memory so there is no history. She cannot really say a complete sentence, so she cannot tell me what she is feeling or thinking. I can speak to her, but she has no clue what I am talking about, so I do not bother telling her about my day. I don't tell her about an interesting patient, a compliment I received or even a tough outcome. I don't get to talk about my goals and dreams for the year. We don't discuss making purchases or improvements to the house. She cannot tell me where she would like to go for dinner, or even what she did that day. At dinner we just sit and eat and stare at each other.

Tonight, what brought this home is that we had a nice dinner (a neighbor brought it by) and cleaned up and we had no plans, and by 7:00 I had done everything that needed to get done. So, we were sitting in our bedroom across from each other and had two hours before her bedtime. I asked her what she wanted to do, and of course she couldn't say anything. I honestly could not think of anything that we could do. There is not much she is able to participate in. I wanted so much to be able to connect with her, but there was nothing. We were made for intimacy and without it, we struggle. Certainly, God can meet that need and He does – especially for those who are single. But when the spouse is still there, but not able to communicate, it is painfully lonely. I find that it even causes me to pull back in all other relationships as well, and I have to be very attentive to stay on top of those or I will just crawl into my shell. Unfortunately, there is no one else that can meet that need.

There is a very real temptation to replace that lost intimacy - often with another person of the opposite sex. It is a subtle temptation, and one that most people do not consciously go out and look for, but it can really sneak up on you. Fortunately for me, my kids and especially my son, understand this and he has been bold to question me openly about this. At first, I was taken back, but then I was so appreciative that he was bold, and that we had the kind of relationship where he felt he could confront me on this issue. Unfortunately, there are also even darker ways to try to meet this need – pornography, adult videos, or even prostitution (and I have seen all of them in my patients). People will try to justify these kinds of behaviors, but they are not acceptable at all. Even Christians can go down this path, so we all need help. I meet with a friend every week, an accountability partner, with whom I share everything, so that I do not even start to walk in that direction. It is a hard subject, but there is nothing easy with Alzheimer's.

Chapter Twenty-Two

Quite A Decade

2018

By now, we had moved into 2018 and it was a mixture of good and bad, which by this time, I had come to realize would be my lot for the duration of this disease. The day after Valentine's, we welcomed our newest grandchild, Wylder Paul Sudan. Yes, it was a son with the last name of Sudan. He has the burden and distinction of being the only one to carry on the Sudan name. I went up to Michigan to welcome him into the world. By this time, I was no longer taking Luana on airplane trips as it was too hard to get her through airports. I went back to Michigan at the beginning of May to do my annual CME course up there at the University of Michigan Medical School. No sooner than after I got back, we welcomed another grandchild on Mother's Day – Sienna Willow – the daughter of Mary Beth and Alejandro. She is the 16th and the last of our grandchildren. It was bittersweet, in the sense that by having two other kids, aged 3 and 1, Mary Beth needed help from her mother. Her mother-in-law lives in Peru and could not help. But neither could Luana. This was the first time where she could literally do nothing to help. With each child, she could offer less and less, but now nothing. We both shed tears over that. On the other hand, even at number 16, the beauty and wonder of grandchildren is still as sweet as ever. It never gets old.

The summer proved to be very busy. Toward the end of July, I flew back up to Michigan, but this time it was to help my son drive the U-Haul from Michigan back to Dallas, where he was to begin a new job working with his brother-in-law remodeling homes. It was good to get him back in Texas. Then, just a few weeks later, I went with a doctor friend of mine back to Uganda for two weeks. This was the first time that I did not take Luana with me and that part was sad, but we had a great trip. By this time, the hospital had been finished and we spent the whole time working there and in the outpatient clinic. We were able to give relief to the missionary doctor there as well as teach the Ugandan equivalent of a PA. We helped them with the assessment and management of patients, but also tried to disciple them in their faith. We worked on some new protocols for the hospital and got to interact with the orphans as well.

Just a few more weeks after that, we made an unforgettable trip to Redding, California, and Bethel Church. It is a trip that I had been wanting to do for years, but never got around to it. A few friends encouraged me to do it, and then all of the kids got behind it, and we made it a family trip, with kids and spouses. Bethel is well known for its healing ministry, and I wanted to take Luana and have them pray over her. We went a day early, got a sitter for Luana, and then did a hike in the Lassen Volcanos National Park. It was so good to do a long hike with my kids and their spouses. It was a little dicey as there was a large forest fire just north of Redding, and there was smoke in the city the whole time we were there. The next day, we took Luana to the healing rooms and they were very nice and respectful and prayed over her. Though we did not receive the physical healing for which we were hoping, it was an amazing time. It was so encouraging to see all of my kids and their spouses joined together in prayer and believing for the miraculous. Words cannot describe all that was in my heart that day.

As Luana was deteriorating mentally and physically, her caregiving needs were growing more and more. By this time, we had already hired an agency and they were coming Monday through Friday for various times throughout the day. This was supplemented by her sister who was still watching her several days a week. Several things forced our hand. It was getting too much for her sister to handle her by herself, so I knew that I needed to have full-time help while I was at work. The agency that we used did a good job, but they had to piecemeal several caregivers to meet our needs. In addition, there was a high turnover, and so we were constantly having to train new people. Plus, it was expensive and would get more so with the proposed increased hours.

Therefore, I started asking around and I heard about an extended family that did caregiving all over the area. I called and set up an appointment with the matriarch. I liked what I had heard and decided to give it a try and her daughter, Stephanie, came to be Luana's full-time caregiver (M-F from 7:30 to 5:30). It turned out to be one of the best decisions I made concerning Luana's care.

She was in her mid-twenties and had just recently gotten married. Shortly after she started working for us, she became pregnant. She was incredibly dependable – always on time and if she ever had to miss, she had someone else already lined up, usually one of her many cousins or her sister. In fact, one time she even showed up when she had the flu and I had to convince her that she needed to go home. I cannot tell you how comforting it is to have a caregiver that you can count on. But more than just dependable, Stephanie truly cared about Luana. She was kind and compassionate toward her. Even after Luana ended up in the memory care facility, Stephanie would go by and see her from time to time. And now, she will still text me on occasion to ask how we are doing. The third thing, besides being dependable and caring, was that she did an excellent job. She knew what she was doing and was able to push Luana to do what she could do, but knew what she could not.

By that fall, she had given birth and I decided to take a risk. I kept her on board and let her bring her baby with her. It turned out to be a great decision and was a win–win situation. I was able to keep her as a caregiver, and the baby did not get in the way, and in fact, it was good for Luana as she loves little babies. At the same time, she got free child care from the best person available. Moving forward, she ended up getting pregnant again and worked until almost delivery time for the second child and this was one of the reasons down the road that led us to the memory facility.

One of the interesting things about Alzheimer's is that even though it is a disease affecting cognitive function, it eventually affects the patient's motor skills as well. It is of course later in the disease process, but it was really hitting Luana at this time. Her walking got slower and slower and more and more unsteady (though fortunately she never fell). By this time, I got her a wheelchair, mainly to use when we were out, and she had to walk long distances – like to church or a ballgame. It was amazing how much better it was having the wheelchair. I had always thought of them as cumbersome, but once you get the hang of it, you can get it in and out of the car quickly and you can get to places so much quicker than with her walking. As a corollary to getting a wheelchair, I had to apply for and get a handicap sticker. That was a little hard for me emotionally, as it really showed me the reality that we were handicapped. Because she could not walk well, I had stopped going to the Baylor sporting events which was something that I loved doing (and it was a fun outing for Luana as well). The addition of the wheelchair allowed me to go to the baseball games as they were very much wheelchair-friendly. Sadly, the basketball arena is not, and so I still could not take her to those; nor to football.

Two other medical issues were going on at this time as well. One, which I briefly mentioned when we went on a trip to Uganda, was her passing out spells. Medically, we call these syncopal spells. Over several years, she has had a half dozen or so of them. These are not related to her Alzheimer's and though we did some evaluation (not an extensive one as I did not feel there was much reason in light of her severe Alzheimer's), we never did find the cause. She even had a few after moving to the memory care facility, which caused quite a stir there as you can imagine.

The other problem was seizures. These can be a result of Alzheimer's (in 10% of patients) and are a late occurrence. The first one happened over Thanksgiving the year before and I will never forget it. We were at my daughter's house in Dallas, and we were asleep when I woke up to the shaking of the bed. I looked over and saw Luana in a full-blown grand mal seizure. I did the usual things – turned her on her side, made sure the airway was clear and waited until it stopped. I had to change her pajamas and put towels over where she had wet the bed. She was post ictal and so stayed asleep, but I laid there until morning, not being able to go back to sleep. Now, as a physician, I have witnessed hundreds of seizures and am not scared of them, but I can tell you that it is a lot different when it is your wife and wakes you up from a dead sleep.

I did not take her to the ER and did not even take her in to get it evaluated. Even if we found something, I was not going to do anything to treat it. I decided against putting her on medication since she was already having trouble getting her meds down. Since then, she has had a seizure about every 4-5 months. They have all been at night and I am about as used to them as you can be with seizures.

To summarize where we were at this point in the journey, I am going to get help from two blog posts. One was at the beginning of the year and described where she was in her ability to do her

ADLs. The second one was at the end of the year and described how much she had changed just in the course of one year. Looking back over that for me was pretty sobering.

> We have covered a lot of different topics over the past several months. But I thought it was time just to give you an update on Luana. I will start by going through the ADLs since that is a pretty good indicator of how an Alzheimer's patient is doing.
>
> So as far as feeding, Luana has gotten to the point where I am having to feed her about 80% of the time. She can do it at times but then she loses interest and just quits. I now try to order things at restaurants that are easier for her to eat, such as finger foods. Then, of course, I always sit on her right side, as that makes it easier to feed her. As long as I feed her, she eats pretty well, but she does not eat many snacks and only occasionally a dessert.
>
> She cannot go to the bathroom by herself. Fortunately, she is not incontinent (we have dealt with spells of that and it is brutal). She will not tell me when she needs to go, but if I ask her then she will tell me yes or no, so that is helpful. Sometimes when she needs to go (especially #2) she will get a grimace or pained look on her face, and I recognize that and ask her if she needs to go. When we get into the bathroom, I have to help her get her pants

down and her panties down and then she will sit down and go. Then, of course, we cannot forget the cleaning part, and I have to do that as well.

Transferring refers to the ability to get from her chair or bed to the bathroom or the table. She is able to do that without any problems. Though I will say, she is having a harder and harder time getting up. She can walk independently, but she is very nervous about falling (even though she never has) and is super cautious and slow. She can still do the stairs as long as there is a rail and she holds on to that with both hands. When we are walking across a large area, she is so slow, she actually pulls against me when I am holding her hand so that I am literally dragging her along. By the time we get there, my arm is sore from pulling her.

Bathing we talked about recently. She cannot do it at all. I usually give her a bath half the time and a shower the other half. I will fill up the tub and then help her into it. I scrub her and rinse her off. Getting out of the tub is a challenge and I am not sure how much longer we will be able to do that. I then have to dry her off, put on her deodorant and brush her hair. She does not like taking a bath, but so far has not put up any significant resistance.

Dressing is another challenge. I have to pick out her clothes (you are all thinking that that cannot be good for Luana – but I have actually gotten better. I even buy her clothes as well, and my girls have approved of what I pick out. That is in itself a miracle and shows the grace of God.) Each morning I have to take off her pajamas and then put on her clothes. I physically have to put her top over her head and then take each arm and put them through the sleeve. Then to get her pants on I have her sit down and put them over her feet and partially up her legs and then will have her stand up and pull them up the rest of the way. Then I have her sit down again in order to get her shoes on. At night we do the same thing in reverse.

And this is the second one:

Today marks the 10th anniversary of the definitive diagnosis of Alzheimer's for Luana. I remember the day well. I was off and took her to see the Neurologist. He did the typical mental status exam and she did poorly as expected and he gave her the diagnosis which I already knew she had. I brought her home and my kids were all there since it was almost Christmas. I told them the news and there was a lot of sobbing. It is hard to believe it has been that long that we have been on this journey. Actually, it has been longer than that, since I had noticed symptoms for about a year and a half before the official diagnosis. We thought it might be stress, but of course it was not. Interestingly, my daughter was reading one of her journals from 2003 and multiple times she writes a prayer to God to help her think clearly. It makes me wonder if she was experiencing some symptoms as far back as then.

I thought this would be a good time to reflect on where she is in her disease course. Frequently, I am asked by friends and patients as to how Luana is doing. I usually respond by saying that she is about the same, or that she is slowly getting worse as we would expect. But I don't really feel that. It seems like she is about the same day to day. But that is what is so deceptive when you are around someone every day. You do not see the changes. It is like watching your kids grow. You do not see it until you go visit Aunt Betty and she exclaims "Oh my, how they have grown." Or, you see it when they no longer fit into their clothes. The point is that you have to have a reference. So, when I look back to where she was a year ago, I see indeed, that she has gone down quite a bit.

We started the year with her walking (although she had started to slow down), but we end the year with her in a wheelchair most of the time. She can still walk but it is so slow and it requires me literally pulling her to where my arm aches, that the wheelchair is better if there is any distance at all. I used it for the first time this week taking her to church. At the same time, I had to get a handicap parking permit for her. We started the year in the same bedroom we have had downstairs for the past 30 years. We ended the year in the bedroom upstairs (actually it is the street level since it is a split-level house) that we first used when we moved in. This is because she was getting too unstable walking up the stairs. I had anticipated this and had converted our tub into a walk-in shower, so that is helpful as well.

What are other changes? I no longer am able to take her with me grocery shopping. I stopped taking her to the football games as it was too hard to get her there. I have also not tried to take her to the basketball games. In fact, I get out less and less these days as it is getting too hard to get her in and out of the car. I am not sure what I will do when I cannot do that at all. I no longer give her a bath, as she has a very difficult time getting out of the tub. I got a shower chair and a shower hose and bathe her that way. She is no longer able to swallow pills by giving them to her with water. I have to put them on a spoon with her cereal in the mornings.

These are just some of the changes which have taken place just this past year. So, when I look at it from that perspective, I see that she has gone down more than just a little. I try not to speculate, but it does make one wonder where we will be a year from now. Frankly, it is terrifying. Fortunately, through every stage, God has been faithful to give me the strength and patience to handle every situation. Thus, I am not fearful, but I am sad. It is so hard to see her go downhill. It is so lonely to be with her and not be able to communicate. It is like experiencing death every single day. Unless you have been there you cannot understand it. It is the fraternity of caregivers – and I can assure you that you do not want to join.

Chapter Twenty-Three

Children's Perspective

2018

I can't remember what life was like before her disease. It is something that I think is common in these kinds of situations, but it is really distressing. Since by this time, we had been down this road for ten years, I could not remember the way Luana was before it hit. I have a hard time remembering what our life was like and how we interacted. I remember that it was good and we enjoyed being together, but the details are so fuzzy. Why is this? I think one of the reasons is that every day I see her like she is now, and I am constantly reminded of that, and it is difficult to separate the former from the current.

I see this happen with my patients whose loved one has a terminal illness and is ill for several years before they die. It is so hard as they try to take care of them, they are met with the immediate and they, too, have a hard time remembering before the illness. The good news is that, with time, after the patient has passed, those memories begin to come back. I am hopeful that it will be true for me because I want to remember her as she was and not as she is now.

Another thing that I have not discussed, but could have right in the beginning, is the question of genetic testing. It came up recently with my kids as we were discussing it while the "23 and me" craze has been in the news. Here is a post I wrote describing it:

> So, what does this question in the title mean? There has been a bit of controversy in the Sudan family as of late, and it has to do with the question of genetic testing. Some of my children are wanting to get tested to see if they have the "gene" for Alzheimer's. Others are just as adamant not to get tested. The problem is that if one knows it will be extremely hard not to tell the others. So, we really need to all agree on this. When first diagnosed, Luana enrolled in the ongoing research at the Memory Research Center at UT Southwestern Medical Center, as I mentioned earlier. As a part of their research, they tested her for everything, including all of the genetic markers. Unfortunately, they do not tell the subjects the results of the studies, so we do not know. Early on, we also all agreed not to get Luana tested independently. There was little discussion about it then, until recently. All of them are curious of course, since they all have some degree of risk for developing the disease. In addition, the spouses have a highly vested interest in the matter.
>
> So, what is this genetic testing all about? Well, Alzheimer's is generally divided into two basic groups. The smaller of the groups is the early onset Alzheimer's disease (EOAD) which refers to those whose onset occurs generally before the age of 60.

The much larger group is the late onset Alzheimer's disease (LOAD) which then would be those whose onset is after the age of 60. The reason for the differentiation is that EOAD is much more likely to have a determinative genetic defect than LOAD. Without boring you with all of the details, EOAD has three gene defects that are associated with it (APP, Presenelin 1, Presenelin 2). Each of these are autosomal dominant and have a virtually 100% penetrance. All that means is that if you have one of the genes then you are assured of developing the disease. In spite of that, only about 1% of all Alzheimer's patients have one of these three genes; 60-70% of familial EOAD have one of them and 10% of all EOAD patients have one of them. Thus, unless you are one of the familial EOAD, then you are not likely to have one of the genes. For informational purposes, familial AD is where there are three or more people with the disease over two or more generations with two of the others being a first degree relative to the third. So, while Luana has multiple family members with AD, including both grandmothers and several aunts, she does not truly fit the description. Her father lived to be 91 and never had AD so it could not have come from his side. Her mother died early at age 62 and could have carried a gene but lived just beyond the EOAD age so that is not likely either.

What about LOAD? Well, it is much more complex genetically, and probably involves a number of genes with only partial penetrance and a lot of environmental and other factors. There is one gene that has been definitively associated with it. The gene is called APOE4 and it is involved in cholesterol metabolism. Most studies show that if you receive one copy of this from a parent then you will have a 4-fold increased risk of developing the disease. But if you receive a copy from both parents then you have an almost 20-fold increased risk.

Where does that leave us? Since Luana probably does not have the true familial EOAD, her risk of having one of the three genes is only 10%. What are the advantages of knowing if you have the gene? Mind you, that if you do not have the gene, you are not off the hook since 90% of EOAD patients do not have the gene. Well, some people are planners and knowing will really help them plan for the future. It might affect where they decide to live or what job to do, etc. They might want to participate in a drug trial to prevent the disease. So, what are the disadvantages? It can certainly lead to depression, loss of the desire to pursue long term goals, terrible anxiety as to when it will start, believing it has begun every time you forget someone's name. And since there is no really effective treatment and certainly no cure, knowing does not help prevent anything.

What would you do, indeed? Every semester when I taught my class at Baylor University on the topic of aging and I got to the class on dementia, I would pose this question to the students. And every semester, the response was split at almost 50-50. To this day, our own family has not reached a conclusion. I tend to side on the not knowing.

One of the advantages I have is that I have a very involved and supportive family, and I have four children and four wonderful in-laws. But as supportive as they are, they do not really know what all you, as the caregiver, are going through. So, this summer in 2018, they got to experience it first-hand. I will let you read it in the words of my oldest daughter, Christy.

> This spring, my dad started talking to us about wanting to go overseas to Uganda, and a place called Restoration Gateway, where he has served many times in the past. As his children, we of course wanted to make that available to him, knowing that while it would be challenging, it would be a much-needed break for him from taking care of mom.
>
> At first, we discussed possibly putting her in a respite care center, but after thinking about it and talking together, we decided that we weren't ready for mom to have to be in a place like that. So, we decided the best way to handle this would be for us to all tackle watching mom together. We (my family who lives in Michigan) were already going to be in Texas for a conference so I asked my dad if he could make the trip after the conference. That way I would be available to help watch mom.

Initially, I thought I could do it the whole two weeks, but after talking it over with my siblings, my sister Amy and I decided it would be best if we all did it together. To be honest, I was really nervous. I live in Michigan, so I don't see my mom that often, and while my other sisters have taken care of her for a week at a time, I haven't been able to do that for my dad because of where I live. I knew mom's condition had worsened, and has required even more care and I honestly wasn't sure how I would do – or how mom would do with me being the primary caregiver.

The way it worked out was that I had her by myself for the first four days, which as I said, made me very nervous. We were going with my in laws on a short trip and were bringing my mom with us. Fortunately, they also live in Waco and have known mom for years and are very kind to her and very helpful and supportive. Thankfully mom did great with me, and even though she doesn't see me very often, she was very receptive to me.

The first night was rather comical as I gave her a bath for the first time and realized I couldn't get her out of the bathtub. I had to call my sister for backup help as to what to do in this situation. Mom and I just laughed together and so did my sister. But really, I wanted to cry. It was so sad to see how helpless she had become. I also had to get used to putting her in and out of the car, and putting her on the toilet to go to the bathroom. To be honest, it was physically demanding and I hurt my back in the process. Fortunately, it was nothing serious and it is well now, but it made me realize how important good technique is. I am a nurse and know those things, but most of my career has been in pediatrics so lifting was never a problem.

Thankfully after those first few days and once I got the hang of it, things went as well as they could. But I was exhausted after only a few days, and was amazed at how dad did it day in and day out. After our trip to the lake with my in laws, and we were back in town, my sisters and sister-in-law came down and it was a tag team approach to watching mom. That made all the difference. When we did it together, it wasn't one person taking her to the bathroom all the time – we took turns. And we took turns feeding her, and making sure she stayed hydrated since she has a problem drinking enough fluids.

We stayed in Waco for a few more days, and had her usual caregiver come which was helpful for mom (a familiar face and routine), and us because it gave us a little break. Even though there were four of us, there were also 16 kids between me and my three siblings. We realized that it is pretty difficult to take mom places when you have 16 kids in addition to her.

After that, we went up to Dallas and stayed the second week there, and again switched off which house my mom stayed. We all did it together. We hung out at one of my sister's houses and had wild chaotic times with the kids. I realized after finishing the time with mom, how much easier it was once we were all doing it together, and that that is how we were intended to live. God created us to live in the context of community and families, and when you live in this manner, the load isn't as heavy. So, where it would have been a lot for me to take care of mom solo for two weeks, the load was much lighter when we were able to do it together.

I realized that we all have different issues and needs – my encouragement is to not look at something that is hard, as something you can't do, but who can you invite into the situation to carry this load with you. It just takes a little courage and vulnerability to ask for help. It also takes humility, but that is the kind of heart that God is looking for. Having needs puts you in a place to learn these things.

So, there you have it – straight from the heart of my firstborn. And she is a very strong woman, talented, a leader and extremely capable. So, if she needed help, we all do. Along the same lines, I needed help as I was starting to get depressed from the stress and overwork. This is often an overlooked component to the care of Alzheimer's patients, and more specifically to the caregivers. Here is a post I wrote on where I was at the time:

> Depression is widely known to be a problem with Alzheimer's patients and a lot has been written on it, but not much has been written about depression in caregivers of Alzheimer's patients. Now, I am not one who is given much to depression, but it is a common problem. What got me thinking about this, is that I have been somewhat down over the past few days. The proper term would probably be melancholy. Now, it is not uncommon at all for people in general to have short periods of melancholy. That is not depression. The diagnosis is made when there are these kind of days >50% of the time over a period of weeks to months. There are usually other associated symptoms as well. But this post is not about how to diagnose depression. Rather it is to explore all of the reasons why caregivers get depressed, and then to explore ways to prevent it from happening.
>
> The first reason is the emotional impact of seeing your loved one in this condition, especially if it is your spouse. And it is not just an occasional time of going over to a friend's house and seeing how bad they are. They are there every day, all day long, as a constant reminder of what has been lost. Along with that, is the loss of your best friend, the loss of intimacy and sometimes (as is with me) the loss of

any conversation. This leads to a second reason and that is loneliness. Even though there is someone there, there is no real communication. Add to that, is the fact that so many of your friends tend to stay away because they feel awkward around Alzheimer's patients. And to make matters worse, it gets harder to take the patient outside of the home, so you have even less social interaction.

Next comes fatigue and caregivers have fatigue for two main reasons. One, is just that there are so many things to do to take care of the patient as well as the house. The second, is that you often lose a lot of sleep since the patient is often getting up in the middle of the night, or having a hard time going to sleep at all. Fatigue is a common precursor to depression, but it is also a common symptom of depression. Another reason is the constancy of the situation. The patient is always there and you know it is going to go on for years. We are already in our tenth year and I could easily see it going on for another ten years. That in itself is depressing. To make matters worse, you know that it is not going to get better but in fact, it will get worse. This is unlike caring for a little baby who you know will grow and be able to do more and more as time goes on. Related to that, and another source of depression, is the fact that you get no positive feedback, no thank you, no cute little smile.

Another reason, and this is a big one for me, is that you usually have to give up most of your other activities and areas of service and ministry. Thus, you feel that you are worthless and that you are contributing nothing to your church or to society. In essence, you feel that you are on the sidelines and out of the game. I know intellectually that this is not true, but that is how a lot of us feel and that can be depressing.

There are a number of other reasons specific to different individuals, but this gives you a pretty good idea. So, what can the community as a whole and more specifically the small community of the caregiver do to prevent depression setting in? Obviously, there are some things which just cannot be changed. A lot of other things I addressed recently in the series of the role of the church. Most of the things needed involve just being a friend. That would mean not being afraid to interact with the patient and/or caregiver. You could team up with another and have one stay with the patient while the other meets the caregiver for lunch/breakfast. It might mean assisting with chores around the house. For some, it could involve staying over at night to give the caregiver a full night's sleep. The possibilities are limited only by your imagination. If you have a friend who is a caregiver, pray about what God would have you to do.

One other thing that I thought would be interesting, is the concept of trust. When you give care to another person, they have to trust you. This is a hard thing for Alzheimer's patients to grasp, but there are also spiritual lessons for us in this as well and I capture both in this post, and that will allow us to close out the year 2018.

We are in the parking lot of the gym where I work out, headed to the car. It is dusk and I am leading Luana by the hand (actually pulling her as her steps are so short that we would never get there if I did not). When we get to a change in the type of pavement, she pulls back and will not move (even though it is all completely flat). I encourage her to step over it saying "You have to trust me. I would not lead you astray or let you fall." She never does, but we eventually make it to the car.

So, I started to think about trust and Alzheimer's. I began to think how frightening it would be to wake up every day and not know where I was, or what the day held. They have to walk in that darkness every day. So, by default they have to trust a lot of people. I wonder if it is natural, or are some people easier to trust than others, even in Alzheimer's patients? Often, they have to trust people they have never seen before. At least with me, she recognizes someone who is familiar, even if she does not know my name.

So, let's go through a day and see where this trust thing leads. When we first get up, she has to trust that I will dress her in clothes that match (before she became ill, she would never trust me to do that). Then, she has to trust that I am giving her safe and nutritious food. She has to trust her caregiver when they get in the car to go run an errand. She has to trust when we lead her by the hand, when we put her on the toilet and when we give her a bath. It goes on and on, but you get the picture. Trust is an ongoing fact of life.

Then I started thinking that it is really no different for the rest of us. We have to trust people all day long. We have to trust the people who make our food, either at the grocery store or in a restaurant. We trust the people who bring us the news (at least we used to). We trust our doctors, lawyers, plumbers, electricians, roofers and so many others who do things for us. We trust our spouse. Where would we be without trust? We would be anxious and it would lead to dysfunction. It is a root of a lot of maladies.

Finally, I started thinking that this is what God has been telling us all along. "You just have to trust me. I will not lead you astray nor will I let you fall." To trust Him (have faith) is really what Christianity is all about. In fact, the Bible says that without faith (trust) it is impossible to please God. So, why is it so hard to just follow Him without holding back? I think the biggest reason is that we do not truly understand the character of God. If we really knew (not just intellectually, but deep down in our hearts) that God was good, and always had our best interests in mind, then I think we would not pull back. As with people, trust in God is developed over time. As we see Him be faithful, then we learn to trust Him more and more. It is amazing, if you keep your eyes and ears open, how much we can learn from our Alzheimer's patients.

Chapter Twenty-Four

Things I Never Thought I Would Do

2019

The year 2019 would turn out to be a pivotal year for us. At this point, Luana was going downhill fast and I was running out of steam. We had been dealing with this for the past 11 years, and while the first few years were not that bad, the past few have been brutal – physically, mentally and emotionally. Fortunately, I was still doing well spiritually and that was what was really holding me together.

Early in the year, we find out that our caregiver, Stephanie, was pregnant again with her second child. Therefore, I knew that her days helping us were numbered, and that made me sad as she was so good.

Also, I was starting to get depressed, more than just the melancholy that I described earlier. Partly, it was the stress and being overworked. But a large part of it was the loneliness. Physically she was right there, but there was no relationship, since she could not talk or communicate in any reasonable way at all. And, because I could not leave her (it was so difficult by this time to take her anywhere), I spent most of the time at home (when I was not at work). I tend to be more on the introverted side of the spectrum anyway, but I still like people and like being around them, and knew that I needed that fellowship, but could not get it.

Here is an excerpt from a post about being overworked that I wrote in January of that year:

> "Now you go home and get some rest, you hear?" I heard several of my staff say to me last Friday as I was leaving for the weekend, having endured several days of working while sick. I really intended to do just that, and drove home with eager anticipation of lots of rest as we had nothing we really had to do. Then, as I said goodbye to Stephanie, Luana's caregiver, at 5:30 it hit me that rather than rest, I had Lu by myself for the next 62 hours. I thought I would describe what the minimum amount of work required to care for Lu would be in a typical day, and see if rest is in the cards. This will also help me to chart where she is right now, so I will be able to see the changes by this time next year.
>
> I usually get up an hour before Lu, so I can have my Bible study and prayer time. This is very important to me in keeping my heart aligned correctly. Once that is over, I go into the bedroom and wake her up. I immediately take her to the toilet. As she is usually wet, I remover her pajama bottoms and then cut her diaper off. I do that because she also usually has stool in the diaper and if you try to pull it off normally, the poop gets all over her legs. I then don my gloves, and with toilet paper and wipes, clean up her bottom. Next, I put on a new diaper and go back into the room to put on

her pants and socks and shoes, as well as a new top. At this point, we head into the kitchen, though it is not easy as it sounds, since I literally have to pull her all of the way. I then prepare breakfast, which, let's be honest, is nothing fancy – usually cereal. I prepare for both of us with drinks and I get her meds out. But not so fast there – I don't just put the food in front of her and let her eat - I have to feed her every bite. When finished, I clean the dishes and put them in the dishwasher (and run it when it is full). Lastly, I brush her teeth. So, now we are ready to start the day.

Since it is the weekend, we usually have a few free hours, though it is not completely, as I do not like to just let her sit there and do nothing. So, I usually try to bring her close to where I am. Also, during that time, I have to take her to the bathroom a few times, pull her diaper and pants down and encourage her to let her pee out (by this time she was not peeing freely and it took a lot of coaxing).

At noon, we head back to the kitchen and I then prepare lunch – again, nothing fancy, which usually means a sandwich with chips and a drink. Again, I have to feed her every bite and encourage her to drink. When we are finished, I clean up the mess.

After lunch, we again have some free time, though it is stressful for me trying to find something that she can do, rather than just sit there all afternoon or watch TV. Again, there are trips to the bathroom. For dinner, the preparation is a little more involved, but it is the same process and of course, I have to feed her and clean up. We have a little more time after dinner before bed, but I am usually putting in a couple of loads of laundry, then drying and folding.

Before bed, I have to give her a bath/shower (usually every other day). I take off her clothes and get her into the shower and she sits on a shower chair. I use the wand and wet her hair and then bathe her with a washcloth. Then, I rinse with the wand and wash her hair about every other time. We get her out of the shower, and I dry her off with the towel. Then, I will get her into a new diaper and put her into her pajamas. Lastly, I will brush her teeth and then have her get into the bed. Then, finally, I can rest and that is usually about 8:30!

I was able to get away to see my daughter's family in Michigan a couple of times. I went in February just to see them and then again in May for the annual CME conference that I had been going to since they moved up there. The problem was what to do with Luana. I could no longer take her on the plane with me. Stephanie had offered for her family to watch her the whole time, but I did not want to do that. I thought about respite care, but didn't want to look, because the last time I went to visit a memory care unit, after I left, I sat in my car and just wept. Those places were for really old people and I just could not see Luana in there. Fortunately, my kids stepped up again and I dropped her off there in Dallas with them. They tag-teamed to get it done. The biggest problem was her continence issue (more on that later). By this time, she was pretty well totally wheel chair bound, which is amazing when I look back and see where she was just a year before.

One last note not related to this post but which goes along with the last one. I was talking to Stephanie, who started caring for Luana 11 months ago, and we were commenting about how now she requires the wheelchair most of the time, even in the house. She then reminded me, and I did remember when she mentioned it, that when she first started, she was taking Lu on walks around the block 3-4 times a day. That far down in less than a year!

Because she was going downhill, she was able to do less and less for herself, which obviously meant that there was more and more for me to do. This had happened over a period of years and I had adjusted pretty well. But, there were some things that I was not prepared to do, and frankly, things that I never thought that I would have to do. Here is a post related to that:

> I am standing in the middle of the "Intimates and sleepwear" department at Target. Fortunately, there is no one else around, as I am feeling very awkward. My goal is to find some more pajamas for Luana, since she is incontinent most every night and usually wets her pajamas as well. That way I do not have to wash clothes as often. I am not looking for anything really "intimate." Those days are long past. I just want some regular winter pajamas. I am not finding what I want and there is no one to ask. I

turn a corner onto the next isle and whoa – bras and the like – that is not what I want. I have been here before, but always with Luana, even though I was the one doing the shopping. I have even bought her underwear, but again with her by my side. Now, I am pretty comfortable with my manhood, but it is still awkward. I never, ever thought I would be doing this.

I never did find what I was looking for at Target, so I went to Belk and went through the same process and found what I needed. Fortunately, there the pajamas are not right in the same area as the more intimate items. But this is just one more in a long procession of things that I never thought I would have to do. I can rattle them off. I never thought I would have to dress my wife. I never thought I would have to give her a bath. Certainly not have to shave her legs. I never thought I would have to spoon feed her. I never thought I would have to push her in a wheelchair. And of course, the worst is that I never thought I would have to clean her bottom. I could go on but you get the picture.

The question now becomes "What is the next thing that I never thought I would have to do?" It might be having to give her a bed bath. It might mean having to remove and clean a dirty diaper while she is in bed. It could mean having to go visit her in a nursing home. The point is that all of this is new, and as she continues to deteriorate, her needs will grow and I will be forced into new areas that I never thought I would have to do. But in spite of that we do them because they need to be done. And I want to be the one to do them. When I made that covenant with her almost 42 years ago, I said that I was committed for better and for worse, in sickness and in health. I take my commitments seriously.

As I do these things, I am giving up my pride. But as I do them, I learn humility and I learn how to rely on God and I allow Him to teach me true servanthood. He gives me strength when I cannot do it on my own. I am reminded of the verse in Philippians 4:13 where the apostle Paul says "I can do all things through Him who gives me strength."

Another thing that I never thought that I would have to do, was to catheterize her each day to drain her bladder. This was by far the most demanding. Here is how that played out.

If you remember (in prior posts), Luana would not pee despite my pleadings with her and with God. I (and the sitter) had spent hours of time in the bathroom trying to get her to pee, only to have her release it all during the night, including all over her pajamas and the bed linens. I appreciate all of the suggestions people gave. I tried most of them. Well, I felt that God had spoken that He did not help her pee so that I would get the help I needed. So, in trying to be obedient I called one of my Urology colleagues who suggested that I try doing intermittent catheterizations once or twice a day. That way we would be sure her bladder was empty and I would not have to spend time trying to coax her into peeing. She might still be incontinent during the night, but it would be smaller amounts and not soil everything. That sounded like a splendid idea to me. I had actually thought about doing that a while back, but it was nice to have an official sanction for doing it.

That in itself was a confirmation that I had heard God correctly, and was pursuing the right path. That very night (before I had the supplies) I had her in the bathroom once again with no success. I then prayed and told God that I had done what he asked and so there was no reason now to not help her pee (you would be surprised at what you will do or say when you are desperate). Within 5 seconds she started peeing. I was singing praises. At that point, I felt like the Lord said to me: "Which is easier to say – trust me or pee? But that you (me) may know that you can trust me with everything, I will have her pee."

Well, I started to order the supplies that I needed – catheters, sterile gloves, sterile lubricant, betadine wipes – and ran into a minor problem. No one in Waco carries urinary catheters in store, so I had to order them through a local medical supply store. I ordered #22 French catheters and after a delay due to a backorder, I finally got them in a few days. The other supplies I just ordered on Amazon. I was ready for the big day. My daughter, Amy, who is a nurse practitioner was coming in town, so I thought I would wait for her to help me the first time. I had cathed women before, but it has to have been over 30 years since my last time. It's like riding a bike – right? We got everything together and set to work. I was not sure she would allow us to mess with her private parts as she has always been a very private person. We did have to work to get her legs apart, but were able to locate the urethra and get it in – the #22 is fine for an indwelling catheter, but her urethra was tiny and it did hurt her a little. I since have ordered #14 which is much better for intermittent (though much slower at draining). The first time we got out 1200 cc of urine (a normal full bladder is about 300). It had to feel better for her. The next morning, she was essentially dry – such a blessing. The next night was the time for me to try it solo. I was nervous, but it went well and I can do it by myself easily now.

Now we will try a couple of times a day to get her to pee, but we do not stress about it and only give her about 5 minutes. If she goes, then great, and if it is right before bedtime, then I will not cath her. But if she does not go, then it is no big deal and I will cath her. It is so much less stressful. I now can get the catheter in from start to finish in 2 minutes. It still takes a couple of minutes for it to drain because the hole in the catheter is so small, but Lu does not even wince when I do it with the smaller catheter.

It has been a good solution for me as I did not have to get any special training to do it. Others might find it difficult to learn to cath someone, or may be grossed out by the whole idea of putting a catheter into their wife. But desperate times call for desperate measures. Plus, my medical training kicked in and I am able to compartmentalize those types of things.

In June, we planned to take our Sudan family vacation. Since we have 26 people, we wanted a place where we could drive and we chose southwestern Colorado (it was a long 21 - hour drive but we made it). I found a ranch house that could hold all of us and it turned out to be a great trip. There was plenty of room for the kids to play outside. We took several hikes and went rafting and into the town of Telluride. One of the big questions was whether or not to bring Luana. I wrote a post describing my thought process. In the end, we decided to take her and it worked out amazingly well.

In a week or so we are going to do our mostly annual Sudan family vacation. We will gather together (all 26 of us) in dreamy southwest Colorado. We all love nature and the mountains and hiking, so it promises to be a great time. One big question that loomed over the vacation was what to do with Luana. Should we take her or should we leave her here? There were several big questions that would make up the decision. How well would she do in the altitude? What would we do with her when we all go on a hike? Would we be able to get her in and out of the house with the wheelchair? How would she do on the 16 (or 21) - hour drive? Would it detract from me and my vacation? Obviously, there will be plenty of people to help but it will inevitably fall on me the most, to take care of her, as it should. The easy answer would be to leave her here. After all, she will not really know any difference. She does not really enjoy the kids or grandkids anymore and does not interact with them at all. So, what is the point?

I started looking around again at places for respite care. I was a little nervous about it since the last time I did it I cried so much after touring just one place. Then, I was talking to our caregiver about it and she told me that they could watch her the whole time we were gone. This looked like the ideal situation, but I still was not sure. I was praying about it and wanting to do the right thing.

Ultimately, I decided that I would bring her on the trip. This was my thinking. First, I just couldn't do that to her. I knew I would feel guilty the whole time, even though I know that there was no need to feel guilty. More importantly, though, was what kind of message did I want to send to my grandchildren. Did I want them to get the impression that when someone is not completely normal then we can just leave them aside? No, I wanted to instill in them the value that all people are created in the image of God and thus are inherently valuable. They are valuable even if they cannot do anything for us. They are valuable from the moment of conception to their last breath. Thus, we include them, even if it is hard and requires more work. Also, I wanted them to see and feel comfortable around people that may have a disability. They all have been around Lu, of course, and they are really good with her. This will just be one more way to reinforce that in them.

So, plans are underway. We will have to make room for not only her but also her wheelchair, diapers, protective pads, catheter supplies, gloves, wipes – much like for a baby. I have a contact near where we are going to see if there is a person who could sit with her while we go on a hike. If not, I will stay back with her. It is not the way I would wish it to be, but there is nothing about this disease that is the way I would want things to be. In the end, she is my wife, I love her and that's that!

Chapter Twenty-Five

The Move

Late 2019

When we got back from that trip to Colorado, things started moving pretty fast through another door into the unknown. Luana was continuing to go downhill very quickly, and I was getting worn down. I did not really know it at the time, but looking back, it was pretty obvious. By this time, I knew that putting her into a memory care facility was unavoidable, but I didn't know when it would be. I felt like I would just know, although I had worked out in my mind some things that would be the trigger. One would be the point at which I could no longer get her in and out of bed. Another would be if she started getting up or awake at night where I could not sleep. Then, if she began to require 24-hour paid care or two caregivers at one time. And then, of course, it would be when my own stress level got too high. Here is an excerpt from a post I did on this in July of that year (2019):

> But in addition to these overt symptoms, stress has a more subtle effect on our bodies. It tends to lower our immune defense system and make us susceptible to all kinds of "real" diseases including infections as well as the previously mentioned chronic diseases. This is certainly difficult to link

directly, which brings me finally to my point in writing this post. Over the past several months, I have had more than my share of illnesses. In April, I had a month of a cough that just would not go away no matter what I did. Then in May, I had my first ever episode of vertigo. While in Colorado, I fell and sustained a high ankle sprain. Then a week later, I had my first ever attack of gout. And now, I am dealing with another two-week (so far) cough and bilateral conjunctivitis. Now, these may all be coincidences, but I am starting to think that it might be signs of stress. I am certainly not naïve enough to think that I don't have stress. Anyone who is a caregiver has a tremendous amount of stress, and all are at risk of getting sick.

So, I have been evaluating my situation and have spoken with my children and am making changes to try to reduce the stress level. Of course, there is just so much you can eliminate, but any little bit helps. In addition, maintaining a regular exercise program can help and I have always been proactive about that. If you are a caregiver, you need to pay attention to your own body and seek help if you are having symptoms. We are not invincible.

Mentally I was trying to prepare for it. Putting your loved one in a facility is such a guilt trip. I had long ago given up the idea that I would never do it. But to actually do it is gut-wrenching. There was actually a confluence of several things that really got the ball rolling. One was the situation with our caregiver. She was about to deliver her second child and would no longer be available, as I had mentioned earlier. The second thing was that I had pulled my back for the third time in the past few months trying to lift her. Normally, I have a pretty strong back and have never had any problems, but she was becoming dead weight, and at times even worse, as she would actively fight against me moving her. The third thing was that my oldest daughter, who is a real activator, was in town. She assessed the situation and suggested that we at least look into places. We made some calls and went looking. I was not looking forward to this at all, since I had done it once before and hated it. Thankfully, my daughter was there to go with me. We went first to this memory care facility, and amazingly, we both really liked it and both thought that we could see Luana living there. That was a huge mental shift.

At this point, we called in the backup troops. We wanted this to be a joint decision with me and all four of my children. We called and two of them were able to come down a day or two later. They both were in agreement that this was a good fit. Then my last daughter came down the next weekend, and her approval sealed the deal. I signed the contract and we set a move-in date – September 20. At this point, we were in mid-August and my other daughter had gone back to Michigan and the September date was when she could get back down. They all wanted to be a part of moving her in. Here is my post on my thoughts at the time of making that decision.

> I knew it was coming. It was just a matter of when. In fact, I knew it was coming 11 years ago when this whole thing started. I wanted to put it off as long as I could. In fact, I even prayed that the Lord would take her before I had to make the decision. But alas, that was not to be the case. The decision,

of course, was when to put Luana in a facility. Even writing about it is hard. But I made the decision, and now my life will be forever changed.

So how did we get here? I will try to outline my thoughts and reasoning, not that I need to defend my decision, but hopefully it will be helpful for others who have to make the decision down the line. I have been in and around nursing homes and memory care facilities for the past 35 years. For the first 25 years I would have said dogmatically that I would never put a loved one in one of those. Then 10 years ago after my mother's stroke which left her demented, I had to make that decision to place her. It was difficult, but fortunately, my brother and sister were very supportive. That was at the same time as the early years of Luana's disease. I knew right then that I was eventually going to have to make that decision again.

Fast forward 10 years and as Lu has gotten progressively worse, it became obvious that the time was getting nearer. Several things happened in a short period to bring it to a head. One was my own health (see recent post). I know that stress can affect one's health and I have had a number of health problems this year. My children have been concerned about me. Then over the past month I have hurt my back three times lifting Lu into the car and at other times. Fortunately, it got better in a day or two each time, but I knew that the big one was coming any day and once my back went out then I was in no way going to be able to care for her. On top of that, our sweet caregiver, Stephanie, is about to have her second baby, and so, she was no longer going to be caring for her (in fact today was her last day). Thus, the timing for making the decision was right. I started talking to my kids about the idea and my oldest daughter, who is a real activator, says that we need to go and look at some places. We did and one thing led to another and here we are.

But there were some other things that went into the decision. One was the recognition that Luana just sat around in the kitchen or living room all day, every day. It was not a problem with the caregiver (or me), but just the fact that she cannot do anything. After visiting the facility and seeing that she would be around other people (which she likes), and that there were lots of activities going on (realizing that most of which she could not participate in), I came to the revelation that the facility actually could be better for her. That was an emotional blow. The second emotional blow was admitting that I could not do it all by myself.

At the same time, the questions start running through my mind. Am I pulling the trigger too early? Am I being a wimp by not continuing on? Am I just being selfish? Intellectually, I know the answers to those questions are no, but I cannot keep them from coming into my mind. And then there is the question as to whether I can actually take her to that place and drop her off and leave. The thought just haunts me. Fortunately, my children have been incredibly supportive. They have all come and seen the place and like it, and even though they would rather not have to do this, they understand that it is time. Amazingly, right now I feel a real peace about the decision. I have been praying for direction from the Lord and I think that is a reflection of those prayers. Also, everyone I have talked to has been affirming in my decision. I guess you never know whether it ultimately is the "right" decision, but I feel that as best as I can discern that it is the correct move.

As the day (Sept 20) approaches, I know I will get a lot more emotional about it. I got married a week after I graduated from college, so I have never lived by myself. Life will be forever changed. I will be lost and aimless for a while. I know I will adjust, but it is just so hard to picture. For the past 11 years I have thrown everything I have into trying to care for her and be honoring to her. I am tired and worn out. If there were no other options, I would press on as long as I could stand. To this point, I have no regrets. I just hope I can say the same a year from now. Pray for me during this next month.

Sometimes these decisions are fairly sudden, and you do not have a lot of time to think about it. But I had a little over a month to prepare mentally and emotionally. It was an emotional roller coaster. Especially difficult were the last weeks, since I knew each thing would be the last time she did something. I wrote a post on this as it really made an impact on me.

I was pulling out of the drive at our lake house on Labor Day, leaving after a long day of finishing a shed I had built and fixing a water leak, when it hit me that this would likely be the last time that Luana would come to the lake house. It was particularly meaningful, since the house has been in our family for 32 years. Luana's dad bought it shortly after his first wife (Luana's mother) died. All of our kids grew up there during the summers – swimming in the lake, tubing, water skiing, birthday parties (we have lots of summer birthdays). Now, our grandchildren are doing the same.

Then, it dawned on me that now that we had a firm date to move Luana to the memory care center, there were going to be a lot of last times. Mentally I started to count them off. Last week was her last time to be at lifegroup. This Sunday will be her last time to go to church. The next day will be the last dinner with her sister and her husband. I had taken her to Dallas this weekend and realized that it would be the last time she would go there. Then there will be others – last time to bathe her, to cath her, to put her to bed, and more. Of course, the last and hardest will be the last night she stays at our house, which will be the last time we sleep together. And that, after 42 years of being together. My eyes are tearing even as I write this.

Not everyone has this kind of experience. People who die usually do so either suddenly with no preparation or slowly but not really knowing exactly when, and so the last times are not really obvious. Or, if someone is moving into a facility, it is usually fairly sudden such as after a fall and a hip fracture, or within a few days of making the decision, so there is not much time to contemplate these things. But I will have had roughly four weeks since my decision till she actually moves in. Therefore, I have had a lot of time to think about the decision and all of its ramifications. One of those things is what it will be like to live by myself. What will that be like? What will I eat? Will I cook? Which bed will I sleep in?

I am typically not a very emotional guy, but my emotions have been like a roller coaster these past few weeks. I am also not big on change (I have lived in the same house and had the same job for 34 years, so you get the picture) and this whole process has been difficult. Thankfully, my kids have been rocks for me during this time. They have been sweet to keep their own emotions away from me to try to protect me (though they talk and Marco Polo each other often and I am glad they have each other). So don't be surprised if you are with me and I begin to mutter under my breath "This will be the last time…"

We made the move and it went amazingly well. My kids were rock stars in how they handled the situation and took care of me. I am so thankful for a family that loves each other and loves God. Here is my post on how it went down.

Well, we got Lu moved into the memory care facility on Friday as the culmination of a very difficult week. There were more tears and laughter than I have experienced in a long time. Today, I have been exhausted and I think it is just due to so much emotional energy expended.

The week started much like any other. Work was very busy which was somewhat of a blessing, as I did not have much time to think about what was coming. Wednesday night was our last Lifegroup meeting for Luana and they honored her well. That in itself was emotional but sweet. The next day, all four kids came into town and we met for lunch at one of our favorite restaurants. Then, the girls took my credit card and headed off shopping to get things to decorate her room. That is always scary, but really, they are pretty good about looking for bargains.

That night was a really sweet time for our family. We ate dinner provided by a sweet friend and then just sat around the kitchen table for a long time talking (Be on the alert for a later post on the kitchen table). We then moved to the living room and had a beautiful time of worship and prayer. There was a flood of tears as we just let our guard down, and all of our emotions came out. I then took Lu and did my last catheterization and put her to bed. When I had finished, I just sat on her bed and cried as I thought about this being the last time she will sleep in our home. We then retreated downstairs and watched some home videos, and it was a good time of remembering and a lot of laughing. It was such a good time for all of us.

The next morning, I went to work while the kids went to the facility to fix up her room. They are all very capable and work together very well and the room looked so cute – probably the cutest room in the facility. At noon, I left work and went home to get Luana. I said goodbye to our sweet caregiver and got Lu ready to take her to the facility. Again, I sat down next to her realizing that it was the last time she would be in our home where we have lived for 34 years. I just sobbed. Finally, I composed myself and got her into the car and drove to the facility. They had been ready for her and had a sign out in the lobby saying welcome to Luana Sudan. We took her to her room and then spent several hours with her to help her (and us) get adjusted. Lu took to it well as I knew she would, as she is so laid back and doesn't let much upset her.

We left and were too spent to do much, so we decided to take in a movie. We watched Overcomer which was very good but it was a tearjerker, so we ended up crying more. We then went out to eat. When we finally got home, we were all exhausted emotionally, so we went to bed early. All in all, I felt that it went about as well as it could. Ironically, the next morning I spoke at a caregivers' conference. I had accepted the invitation to speak about 8 months ago and did not want to bow out at the last minute. It ended up going very well and I am glad that I did it.

So, the deed has been done. I am still not sure how I feel. It will be a new normal and it will take time for me to figure out a rhythm for how to love her there. Through this week I have been blown away by all of the love and support that we have received from family and friends. I want to thank all of you who sent cards, brought flowers, made dinner, sent texts, prayed and expressed your love for us all.

Once the move was made, there were a lot of emotions and situations that I had to deal with almost all at once. First there was the emotional aspect of putting your spouse into a long-term care facility. Then there was the guilt that goes along with that, and I have briefly mentioned that already. On the good side, there was the physical relief of not having to care for her daily. Along with that is the relief of the stress that accompanies caregiving. I didn't realize what a toll it had taken on my body until about 2-3 months later, when I started thinking about how much better I was feeling and how much more energy I had. The other aspect is the extreme loneliness that ensues, and then adjusting to life as a sort of single man. Here is a post I wrote related to that idea.

> As long as Luana was living in the house with me, even though she could not really communicate, I never thought of myself as single. She was there, visible and present and I never had to deal with the things that go with singleness. But now that she is in the memory care facility, I am living at home, alone and for all the world look and feel like I am a single man. But of course, I am not – I am still married with a wife, only she does not live with me. We are separated, though certainly not in the sense of the present day use of the term. It is a very strange feeling. I am not yet sure how to navigate this road.
>
> What brought this to mind was an interaction this past week at lifegroup. We were discussing the upcoming events at our church and one of them was an engagement class. Our lifegroup is all 55 and

over and we are all married except for one guy who lost his wife to cancer a few years ago. We all laughed and joked that none of us needed the engagement class, but then looked at this guy and said "unless Joe is going to need it". He promptly looked at me and said that I might as well – but then stopped himself as he realized that I was not actually single yet. It brought home a stark reality. I look and act like I am single (in the sense that I live by myself and go everywhere by myself), but I am not.

I am going to piggy back this discussion onto one about intimacy. I have discussed this to a degree in a past post, probably a year or two ago. But it has really come up for me more since Luana has been in the facility. Intimacy (and here I am not talking about the physical part though that does come into play as well, but the close emotional connection with a spouse) is one of the most important benefits of marriage. It is a very important part of a marriage, and is a near critical need of being human. I say near because there are obviously many men and women who are truly single and doing well. The problem with people in my situation is that there is no legitimate way to solve the problem. It is not like I can go on dates or even have intimate conversations with other women.

But that is what I am really missing right now. I miss sitting down with Luana after work and discussing my day and hers. I miss telling her about interesting patients. I miss being able to talk about our children and our grandchildren and boast to each other of their little achievements, or to be concerned together if there are problems. I miss being able to talk about world and local events and to plan for things in the future. I miss going out to eat with her and sitting with her at ballgames. I miss how I could give her one look and she knew what I meant – I was known by her. I miss being loved by her.

That is all gone and will never come back. And until she passes on, I will never have it. I understand that, but it is still hard. That is also what makes my visits to her so hard. I long so much to sit with her and to just talk and share all of life with her. But she just looks at me and there is nothing there. Fortunately, as a believer, I know that I am known by Him and I am loved by Him. That is helpful, but the human element of intimacy is still missing. So, I function most of the time as if I were single…only I am not.

As I have said all along, God has been incredibly faithful to me every step of the way. He either gives me the strength or the patience I need to deal with Luana, or sometimes He will give someone a word for me. Sometimes He gives me an encouraging word. During this transition period when I was sad for and about Luana, an amazing thing occurred. I wrote a post about this which I think will be encouraging to us all.

I don't know how you feel about hearing from God. I came from a church tradition that taught that we heard from God when He speaks to us in His word. I wholeheartedly agree with that. But over the past 18 years I have been learning that He also speaks to us in many other ways. It is certainly Biblical. God spoke to Elijah in the still small voice, Isaiah tells us that we will hear a voice behind us saying "this is the way, walk in it", Paul heard God speak to him many times and Peter hears Him in a dream. I am not talking about hearing the audible voice of God, but just that quiet voice in your mind. I am not trying to get theological but just prepping you for what is coming.

The other morning, I awoke with a text from my daughter saying that she was praying for me and that she had a word from the Lord. That is not unusual as I have wonderful children (and in-laws) and they pray for me and will occasionally text me a word or a Scripture. This time, she sensed that He was saying that He was restoring my soul. She went to Psalm 23 and felt the whole passage was for me. So, I scratched my usual quiet time that morning and opened my Bible and read Psalm 23 in a fresh way, as if He was speaking directly to me. Interestingly, the phrase that stuck out to me the most was "Thy rod and thy staff, they comfort me". I started thinking about the staff and it was not for comfort – it was used to strike the sheep to keep them moving in the right direction. So how was that a comfort to David. I think he meant that he took comfort in knowing that God was looking out for us, and if we ventured away from where He was leading that He would bring correction (a strike, or maybe some form of suffering). I thought, yes that is comforting, even if hard.

Then I thought about my situation and the suffering that I have been through in our journey with Alzheimer's. I spoke to the Lord and told Him that I certainly can see that He has led me to a good path and a deeper relationship with Him through my suffering. And for that I am eternally grateful, even in my suffering. But then, I asked Him why Luana had to suffer so for me to draw closer to Him. That is when it all started. The Lord spoke to me as clearly as I have ever heard Him in all my years as a believer. He said, "Artie, Luana is not suffering. And I am speaking to her in ways that you can never know." At that point I just lost it. I started crying like a baby with tears just streaming down my face. I didn't even bother to wipe them off. It was such a relief and an encouragement to know that she was not suffering, and that He was speaking to her. Joy flooded my soul. But that was not the end.

I then asked the Lord what He was speaking to her. He said, "She has accomplished everything that I had called her to do and her prize is before her." Again, I was blown away but not surprised since that would certainly fit Luana. So, then I asked what other things He said to her, but at that point He told me that that was not for me to know. And I was totally okay with that. At this point I was totally immersed in my conversation with Him, so I then asked about my suffering and whether it will come to an end. His next comment was piercing, "Do you want me to take her out of the special relationship that we have?" By that, I took it to mean either by healing her or by death. I was too stunned to ask more for a while. Then I asked again about the end for me, but He was just silent.

As I was continuing to meditate on the Psalm, I went back to the beginning where he talks of the Shepherd leading him to green pastures and quiet waters and restoring his soul. So, I asked Jesus about this and said that I felt more like I was in a desert and not lying in green pastures. Then, He said one last thing to me, "Sometimes in order to get to the green pastures you have to cross through deserts. Do not be afraid as the green pastures are coming, they are up ahead and it will not be long." I don't know what that means or what it will look like, but again it was so encouraging.

I am so thankful that I serve a God who cares enough about me, a nobody in this big world, to speak to my daughter who would in turn speak to me and then reveal these words of encouragement. He can and will do the same for you. Listen and ask!!!

The difficult year of 2019 was coming to a close. At the beginning of that year, I never would have dreamed that we would be where we were at the end. I was adjusting to a new normal. Luana was continuing to deteriorate, such that I was glad that we had made the move when we did. This year was to be our turn for Christmas. We debated about where to have it and what to do with Luana. In the end, we decided to have it at our house (which was the first time there in a long time) and we took Luana out of the facility for the day to be with us. But we also had a fun night on the 23rd where we rented out the theater at the facility and brought Lu and all of the grandkids. We watched a movie and ate popcorn and had snacks. It was such a fun night and a good way to honor her.

One of the things you always have in the back of your mind when you move your loved one into a nursing facility is whether you pulled the trigger too soon. It may not be logical and I have had multitudes of people tell me that I did not, but it does go through your mind. Well as things have turned out, I do not think that any more.

Luana had gotten progressively weaker over the past couple of years (remember the picture of her in a recent post where just 2 years ago she was walking independently) such that she went from walking easily with a little support to requiring more support and, by the time we moved her, she was barely walking a few feet with a lot of help. It was getting more and more difficult for me to get her to the bathroom, get her dressed and get her into the bed.

Well now she is to the point where I can barely get her to stand at all. When I go to visit her, I usually try to get her to stand and walk a little bit in order to keep her muscles working. But over the two months that she has been there, she has deteriorated to where I do not even feel safe doing that on my own. I don't know if this is just her natural deterioration or if it is because they do not get her up as much as I did at home. At any rate, I realize that there is no way that I could care for her at home by myself. And if we had a caregiver, then we would need two, at least in the morning to get her up and dressed and at night to do the same and to give her a shower. So, while I am disappointed that she has deteriorated further, I am pleased that we made the decision when we did.

It is difficult to know what will happen next. What will be the next thing to go? She is so far down that there is not much else to lose. She needs full help on all of her ADLs. I think the next big decline step will be when she starts having trouble swallowing. So far, she does not get choked at all and swallows well. But that is a common problem with Alzheimer's patients. We have already decided not to place a feeding tube should she lose the ability to swallow without aspirating (which I think is the right decision for 99.9999% of Alzheimer's patients who get to this point), and so that would mark the beginning of the end. But that might not happen for years. Who knows?

That is one of the biggest problems with Alzheimer's patients. As they deteriorate, you continually have to readjust your expectations, your level of care needed and your own ability to care for them. On a more positive note, I am getting adjusted to life with a spouse in a nursing facility and when and how much to visit. It is not as easy as I thought it would be. And that does not even include the emotional turmoil that you go through. The more I deal with this disease the more I learn.

Christmas 2019:

This was our year to all be together for Christmas and after some back and forth we decided to have it here in Waco. Thus all 24 of them (my four children and their spouses and all sixteen grandkids) descended on Waco and more specifically, my house. So, for a whole week we had 25 people (including me) staying at my house. Now you may think that that sounds like chaos – and you would be right. But it was a good chaos. Amazingly, everyone stayed healthy the whole week and most everyone slept well (we spaced the kiddos out better this time). Fortunately, they all love each other and get along so well that other than a few minor sibling spats (who stole my gum?), there were no real conflicts. And of course, the adults all get along really well so there was no conflict there. The girls did a great job cooking and sharing the load so that we only ate out two times.

The Delaney, where Luana lives, has a theater room which we reserved and we all gathered there on the 23rd to watch "Star". My son-in-law's sweet sister provided a candy bar and we popped popcorn and ate pizza. We brought Luana over and we all had a great time. On the 24th we brought Luana home (for the first time since she moved away – she showed no signs of recognition) and she was with us the whole time as we did our annual cookie decorating contest, and then went with us to church for our Christmas Eve service. After that, we took her back and all of the grandkids come and they sang Christmas carols to the patients there. They did a great job and the patients and families loved it. Then, on Christmas morning we went over there to get her again to bring her home (with two of us it was not difficult to get her into the car). She watched us open gifts (though really, she slept through most of it) and then ate our Christmas meal, before we took her back later that afternoon. She did well throughout all of the comings and goings.

Since Christmas is over, I have gotten back into somewhat of a routine where I go to see her about 4-5 days out of the week. I usually stay anywhere from 30 minutes to an hour. Since most of the time she barely registers that I am there, and of course she cannot talk, there is not much to do. Hence my original question – is it really worth it? Is it worth the effort and time to go out there and sit there? Was it worth the effort to bring her home over Christmas, even though she had no meaningful interaction with the grandkids? I think those are legitimate questions. I will take the two questions separately since they have two very different answers.

The first, whether it is worth my time, is a yes. I do not think it makes any difference to her, but it does to me. I still love her and just getting to see her does something to me. Then, the times when she is more alert and smiles are very precious. I really like when she will make one of her facial expressions that she used to do all of the time – those are the times when I see the old Luana come through. I don't stay long as it does not do either of us any good, but I still need those visits to see her and hold her hand.

The second is tougher. Why put out all of the effort to bring her home to the holiday events when she does not interact at all? The grandkids are sweet to her and say hi and will give her a hug, but then do not spend any other time with her. What is the point? This goes back to when we took her with us all of the way to Colorado this past summer. I think in so doing we are making a statement to our grandchildren. Actually, several statements. One is that not everyone is perfect, and that is okay, and we can still love them and be around them. Another, is that there is value in human life even when we cannot see it and when we get nothing in return. These lessons are worth all of the effort. So as long as we can, we will continue to include her in what we do.

Chapter Twenty-Six

Quarantine

2020

The year 2020 was supposed to be the year of perfect vision – clarity – everything was supposed to come into focus. Well, we all know how that turned out. But in those early days and months, nobody had a clue as to what was coming.

By this time, I was trying to find my rhythm as to when to see Luana and for how long. What was I supposed to do while I was there? How could I best advocate for her? This was a totally different ballgame, and I was surprisingly unprepared. I had been in nursing homes for 35 years in my work as an internist, but it is completely different from the standpoint of a physician and that of a spouse. I try hard to not pull my physician card when dealing with the staff there, unless of course it is an emergency. I try to be super nice to them as they are the ones caring for her, and I feel like they will be more attentive to her if I treat them with courtesy and kindness. As a Christian, this is what I should do anyway.

At the same time, I was dealing with the guilt feelings that are inevitable when you place your spouse in a facility. It is a terrible mind game. I knew intellectually that it was the right decision, but there were always doubts that came up that I had to deal with. To this day, I still wrestle with this question. I wonder, if she could think clearly, would she understand my reasonings and agree? Or would she be furious and feel betrayed? The bottom line is that we will never know, but you have to make a decision one way or the other, and live with the consequences.

My routine that I developed was to go right after work (the facility is a straight 5-minute drive from work and a 7-minute drive from home), and I stayed about 30-45 minutes. I did this five days a week (I took Wednesdays and Sundays off). When I could get off in time, I would try to get there in time to feed her. I did this for two reasons. I could ensure that she would get a full meal. She is a good eater and will eat everything on her plate, but she is slow, so you have to work at it a long time. The staff are good about feeding her, but they do not have the time that I do when I am there, and frequently will stop feeding her before she is finished. The other reason is that it gives me something to do with her when I am there. Since she cannot talk, it can be very difficult to find something to do with her for 45 minutes.

Also, while I was there, I wanted to be a part of the family. And that is really what the unit was. Other family members were also there during meal time and I got to know them. Several were regulars and we would visit since it was hard to communicate with the patients. I did get to know all of the patients as well. I tried to engage the staff and get to know them personally.

Because she was in the facility, I was not tied down and thus I was free to travel. In February, I went to Michigan to see my daughter and her family. We had a wonderful time. Little did I know that it would be the last trip I would take for a good while.

Also in February, our family was hit with a bombshell. My six-year-old grandson was diagnosed with ALL (acute lymphoblastic leukemia). This is a difficult situation for any parent, but especially hard on moms. It is also the kind of situation where those moms need their mom for emotional and physical support. With Luana unavailable due to her illness, my daughter had a much more difficult time with it. Fortunately, she had her siblings and a very good friend network which helped her through those early days. It rocked our world as you can see in my post on this at the time:

> Luana's mother died at the age of 64 (our age now) when Lu was only 32 due to a short bout with lung cancer (yes, she was a smoker). For years after that, I would come home and find her crying randomly. When I would ask her, she would tell me that there was something that happened (good or bad) that she wanted to tell her mother and get her advice, but obviously could not. I could understand it at some level intellectually, but I could never understand it from an emotional or a heart level. My mother was still alive, but also calling her about something with the kids was not anything I did. Ironically, our daughters are experiencing the exact same thing, though at an even younger age and it is even more difficult because she is actually still alive, but not able to meet that need.
>
> This pops up periodically with our girls and I understand it a lot more now. I have tried really hard to be there for them to help in any way that I can – birthday and Christmas gifts, going to their parties, attending sporting events, babysitting – but this is one area where I cannot replace Luana (actually there are many areas). I acknowledge this to them and tell them I understand, and I do not feel slighted or unappreciated – there are just some things that only a mom can do.

This past weekend was one of those events that highlights this problem, and it did so in a big way. On Thursday, my six-year-old grandson started having abdominal pain and he ended up in the ER at Children's hospital in Dallas. After a number of tests, it was determined that he actually had an acute leukemia (ALL – Acute Lymphoblastic Leukemia). He was seen by Oncology and admitted to the hospital. Over the next 24 hours he had a port placed for IV access, a bone marrow biopsy, a spinal tap with intrathecal chemotherapy given, an echocardiogram and then his first dose of systemic chemotherapy.

Needless to say, this is a traumatic event for anyone but especially for a young mother. The most primal and natural response is to call her own mother, to lean on her and cry with her. I felt helpless. My anger at Alzheimer's burned more than it has this whole time. She needed Luana and Luana was not there to console her. And there is no way that I could fill those shoes. To make matters worse, her sisters who were certainly there for her (thank goodness for sisters), also felt the same grief as my daughter and they too needed to talk and process this whole thing. And lastly, I too wanted so much to be able to talk about it with her and hold her hands and pray for them like we used to do in those kinds of situations.

Moms are special. They are irreplaceable. It is how God designed the universe to work. Sin breaks in to destroy this bond in a variety of ways. Fortunately, He does not leave us helpless – He sends other godly women to step into the lives of those who have lost theirs. But He also is our comforter and we can call on Him and fall into His arms and cry on His shoulder. And lastly, His church steps into the gap and provides comfort to the hurting. How thankful we have been for our church which has stepped up in a big way, along with countless friends, neighbors, co-workers and others. Without them, we would have been crushed.

Fortunately for my grandson, his prognosis is still good and we are hopeful and praying for complete healing. But it is a long road and many potential pitfalls. He has had an amazing attitude for which we are incredibly thankful.

He got chemotherapy and as a part of that, high dose steroids, which made his sugar go through the roof. Thus, they had him stay in the hospital that whole first month. He was going to be out of school and he would have to be quarantined. His mom was worried. How do you quarantine a six-year-old? Then hit the pandemic – and the whole world went into quarantine.

For Luana, the lockdown was a whole different matter.

> I guess it is inevitable that I write a post on COVID 19 or the SARS -COV2 virus, since that is what everyone in the world is talking about. It has affected me in a number of ways of which I will get to later, but for the major purpose of this post, the immediate reason is the lockdown in the long-term

care facilities. So Luana, being in the memory care facility, has been in lockdown since 3/13/20 and I have not been able to see her. I have called to check on her and they tell me she is doing fine. Today I even had one of the staff call me and she held up the phone to Lu so I could tell her hello and that I loved her. The person said that Lu got a big grin on her face and that made me happy, but she could also have just said that, knowing that that is what I wanted to hear. Luana did not say anything back but I really did not expect it. One of the remarkable things that has surprised me, is how much I miss seeing her. I really did not think that I would, since when I am there, we cannot talk or have any meaningful communication. But somehow, those short times of just seeing her and holding her hand were doing something deep within me. As I have thought about it, I think that is also the way it is with us and God. Those times we spend with Him each morning do something deep inside of our soul such that when we don't, there is a longing and an emptiness.

I have mixed feelings about the lockdown. I certainly understand the theory behind it, and the impetus for it, which began with the situation with the nursing home in the Seattle area. And the two factors which all nursing facilities have – old patients and close proximity – put them at a particularly high risk. But are we doing them a service to lock out any contact with the very people that give their lives meaning and stability? The administrator's hands are forced due to the media, since any home not doing these measures is "out of touch" and "dangerous". I know I am in the minority here, or at least from anyone who is willing to say it out loud (or in print). For Luana, I do not think it matters that much, because she never knows when the last time I came to see her was, and sometimes hardly acknowledges that I am there when I am there. But for many of these older patients, and especially those with dementia which is milder, that daily contact is vital and its absence can throw them even further off. Many can get irritable and agitated. Since I cannot go in, I have no idea how the residents are really doing.

As the lockdown wore on, I was surprised at how it affected me. I really missed seeing her. I know it seems weird in that she cannot communicate. So what is it that I missed? I'm not sure I can even answer that for myself. Even now, it is the same dynamic when I go to see her. I enjoy being in her presence but when I leave, I am depressed by seeing her in the condition that she is in. Because I was not seeing her, and just coming home from work every day, I felt completely like a single person. I would get even more lonely than I had been. It usually was not evident much until I was getting ready for bed and just lying down, thinking before I closed my eyes. Then it would hit me and I would frequently shed tears. Here is a post on my thoughts at the time when I could not see her:

That is an old and well known saying. I always laugh when I hear it because I always think of my father-in-law who used to make a small change to it and would say to my daughters, his grandchildren, with a wink "Absence makes the heart wander!" Well right now I am experiencing absence (I have not been able to see Luana in almost three weeks now, and no end in sight) and I really do think my heart is growing even fonder. I have been surprised at how much I miss that girl. What has really been interesting is that I am starting to have memories of her back when she was normal. I know that sounds weird – why would you not have those memories? Well, that has been one of my biggest grievances – I have not been able to remember what she was like before the ravishes of Alzheimer's. I think it has to do with seeing someone daily that makes it hard to remember things remotely. But since it has been so long now, some of these are coming back and it is sweet. I have heard that happens when someone dies after a long illness – that you start to remember the good memories and start to forget the recent bad ones.

The other thing I have noted recently is the increasing loneliness. I have experienced it to some degree for years, even when Lu was still in the house, since there was no way to communicate with her. She was there physically but there was no relationship and it was hard. Then, when she moved to the memory care facility, it took on a new level but was still mild and intermittent and I was still able to see her most days of the week. But now that I have not been able to see her, it has really escalated. Certainly, the further isolation caused by the corona virus has aggravated it. Most of the time during the day I am fine, as I am at work and busy and with people. Even when I get home, it is not too bad as I have lots of things to do and am not just sitting around doing nothing. The worst times are late at night when I get into bed and turn out the light and this flood of loneliness sweeps over me. I have spoken with other people who have lost a spouse and they say that is a problem time for them as well. One night recently, it was so overwhelming that I just started crying in my bed. There is no real cure for loneliness.

Despite this, there is a part of it for which I am thankful. I love that I miss Lu – that those feelings are still there, regardless of the lack of positive feedback. I also love that I am getting some memories of her old self. Those make me miss her more but in a good way. And all in all, I am doing well. I am not depressed and I feel well physically and have lots of energy and no lack of things to do. In fact, since there are no sporting events, I have not watched any TV at all. So, I guess my heart will continue to grow fonder.

By the summer, I was getting tired of this and our family had decided we were going to get together regardless. We decided to meet at our lake house since it was more open and we would not be in the big city. It went well over several weekends with different ones. While there one day, I thought about how fun it would be to have Luana with us. I knew that even though she was in a facility, she was not a prisoner there. And since she was private pay and not Medicare, there were no restrictions that we had to deal with. So, I spoke with the director and asked what would happen if I took her out for the weekend? She replied that she would have to be quarantined in her room for two weeks afterwards. I thought that was a good tradeoff, since she does not interact with any of the other residents anyway, and she would not likely know any difference. I discussed it with my kids and they agreed, so we made plans to get together. It turned out to be a big hit and a wonderful weekend. Here is my post on that:

> About a month ago, I was at our lake house by myself enjoying the peace and quiet and the cooler temperature with a gentle breeze, looking out over the lake. I was there to do some writing. While there, I began to think about how much Luana loved the lake house and how fun it would be for her to be able to see it one more time. I then had the thought of taking her out of the memory care facility for a weekend and bringing her with me to the lake house. As I thought about it, there were so many questions that came to mind as to whether this would be possible at all. In view of the COVID crisis, would they even let me take her out? Of course, I am paying for it and she is not a prisoner. So, what would be the ramifications? I suspected she would have to quarantine in her room for two weeks afterwards. Would I be able to handle her?

How would I get her in my car? Once I got there, would I be able to get her out of my car and into her wheelchair? Then would I be able to get her up the steps to get her into the lake house? Would I be able to change her diaper and her clothes by myself?

Very quickly, I realized that I would need help if this was going to happen. So, I floated the idea to my kids in Dallas and they were instantly on board. My youngest daughter agreed that her family would be there when we arrived and she organized the food preparation for the weekend. My son and his family would be there to help with any lifting. The grandchildren started getting excited about seeing Mimi. I spoke with the director of the memory care side of the facility and she thought it was a great idea. She passed it up to her boss who also gave the green light. They said it would require a 14-day quarantine, but I figured it would be worth it, as Luana does not interact with anyone in the facility anyway. So, it was all set and this was to be the weekend. I was nervous all week as to whether we could make it happen. Then, that day came and I was really nervous. I felt like a high school teenager about to go on his first date.

Well, we are back and it happened and it went well – in fact, it was amazing. It was so much better than I could have imagined. I got to the facility right after work and they were ready and had her bag packed. I was able to lift her from the wheelchair by locking my arms around her and then rotating her 90 degrees and sitting her in my car. That was a huge lift, as I then knew I could do the transferring by myself and it took a lot of pressure off of me. We stopped to get a Diet Coke, of course, and then headed straight for the lake house. When we got there (she did great in the car as we listened to a podcast and worship music), my daughter and her family were there. I was able to get her out of the car and into the wheelchair by myself, but it did take two of us to get her up the stairs. I am not sure how much she realized she was at the lake house, as she did not show any special excitement. The kids and grandkids were so sweet to her, even though she did not show any recognition. Occasionally, we would get a smile out of her. Shortly after that, my son and his family arrived, and we sat around and talked and enjoyed just having Luana among us.

My daughter then helped me get her out of her clothes and change her diaper and into her pajamas. It went really smoothly and we put her to bed. I slept in bed with her (for the first time in almost a year) and it went well except at one point she was making all of these involuntary jerking movements like she was about to have another seizure. She did not, however, and for that I was thankful. The next morning, I got up and changed her diaper and got her clothes on all by myself, which I wanted to try to do so that I would know if I could. That was another big milestone. She ate a good breakfast and we put her in a chair out on the deck so she could watch all of the kids playing in the yard and the lake. My other daughter came that morning with her two oldest daughters (the boy is the one with leukemia and could not be around us). Luana did well sitting outside most of the day in the shade, until it got too hot and we moved her back inside. She ate a good lunch and dinner. I got her ready for bed by myself and she had a good night's sleep.

The next morning, I got her up and dressed again and she sat on the deck again as the kids were in the water till lunch, at which time we had to pack up and leave. The drive home was good and we stopped at Bush's chicken for lunch in their drive thru. I stopped briefly at her sister's house to visit with her before taking her back to the facility.

All in all, it could not have gone smoother. There were no clarion moments where she showed recognition, no meaningful words were spoken, no healing happened. But it was so good for all of us just to see her there with us, as we enjoyed each other's company. As I told them afterwards, it was good for my soul. And the other important thing was that I realized that I am able to do it all by myself, so that I can take her home any weekend that I want. I will just have to wait and see how she does in the quarantine, or for the COVID crisis to settle down. It truly was a weekend to remember.

I was also getting antsy about getting out and wanted to do something. I, like most all of us, felt trapped. I have a friend who lives in Maine and is going to PT school. We were tennis buddies and had talked about me going up there to join him and do some hiking in Acadia National Park. At first, it was closed but we kept a close watch on how things were going and when it did open up, we pulled the trigger. I got a flight up there and rented a VRBO near the park. Now Maine was a lot stricter than Texas and I found that I had to either have a negative Covid test within 72 hours or quarantine for 14 days after I got there. The latter was out of the question, so I got my test and it was negative and I flew up there. I met my friend in Portland and then we drove up to the park. We did three full days of hiking and saw most all of the park. It was a glorious time, and we had great weather and good fellowship. It was just what my soul needed.

Over the next couple of months into the fall, I ended up taking her out of the facility for a weekend several more times (about every 4-6 weeks), these times to my home and they worked out well also. She did not seem to mind the quarantine, and it was good for all of us to see her in person. I felt so sorry for those residents, not just in our facility, but in any facility who were not able to get out and in which no one was able to go inside.

As Thanksgiving approached, the family talked about what we should do. It was our turn to be together as a family for this holiday, and we really wanted to go back up to Michigan as we knew my daughter up there was coming home and it would be our last chance to meet there. She loves to host and does an amazing job and was so looking forward to it. We had all bought our plane tickets, but just weeks before the date, the Michigan governor instituted new restrictions such that no more than 10 people in two households could be together at one time. Thus, we restructured our plans and flew them down to Texas. We then had to decide whether to have Thanksgiving in Dallas with one of the kids, or to all come to Waco. The kids all decided that Waco it would be. I was thrilled. Having 25 people in your house for a week could be trying on anyone, but we are used to tight quarters and everyone gets along so well that it works for us. It turned out to be an amazing week. Here is a post about it:

> As with most of 2020, this Thanksgiving was not as planned, but because we were all flexible, we were able to make it a fun time. But it was the first time Luana was not with family on that day. She and I had been together over this holiday for 42 years, but we moved her into the memory facility in September 2019, so she was no longer at home Thanksgiving of last year. That was the year for the in-laws so I was by myself and went down to spend it with my brother and sister in Houston. My daughter Amy's in laws live in the area so she and Blake picked Luana up Thanksgiving Day and she was able to spend it with them and thus not alone.
>
> This year was different – as with all things COVID. Our original plans were to spend Thanksgiving with our daughter in Michigan. This was our year and we were going to all meet up there. Then our daughter, Amy and her family could not make it because her son has ALL and is still on maintenance chemotherapy and his oncologist did not want him flying. Instead, they were going to meet with her in-laws and bring Luana with her as she did last year. The rest of us already had our plane tickets, when the controversial governor of Michigan came down with an executive order that private groups could have no more than 10 people of two families. That ruled us out. We thought

about going anyway, but decided that as believers in Christ, we needed to be obedient to the governing authorities. In an about face, my son-in-law in Michigan was able to get airline tickets and they came down here instead. We decided to do Thanksgiving here in Waco rather than in Dallas. It was such a selfless act on their part, as they were so looking forward to hosting us, since we had never been together as a group in their new home.

The good part about it meant that Amy and her family were then going to be able to join us, and we were going to get Luana out for that day so she could spend it with us as well. Enter COVID once again. It just so happened that one week before Thanksgiving, two people on her wing at the facility tested positive for COVID and all of the others were quarantined in their rooms and all were tested (Luana's test got messed up in transit and we never got results, but she never developed any symptoms). We all discussed it and decided that it would be best not to bring her here and potentially expose everyone. It was a hard decision, but even now I think it was best.

Despite Luana not being there, we had a great time. We did lots of fun family activities, had out annual cookie decorating contest, did our own little turkey trot and then had a marvelous Thanksgiving meal. Everyone stayed healthy, until the night when most people had left and my son-in-law called that he had developed a fever. Over the course of the next week or two everyone came down with Covid except for me and the family with the little boy with leukemia. No one got terribly sick for which we are very thankful. While on the subject, just after Christmas, that little boy and his mother did get Covid (he was asymptomatic) and he gave it to me, which is how I started 2021.

Chapter Twenty-Seven

From Their Lips

2020

Often, I get caught up with my own pain in this journey into the unknown, but it is helpful to stop and realize that I am not the only one who is suffering. There are lots of people who love Luana, and each one experiences the tragedy in different ways. I had each of them write a post on their thoughts and feelings and I am including those from my four children. The first is from my oldest daughter, Christy:

> When I think about this, it is hard to think of how it has impacted me in just one way. It has been such a long road as I have been working with her diagnosis emotionally, and it has affected me in different ways in different seasons. I remember that the time when she first started having worsening symptoms was during my youngest sister's wedding.
>
> We were eating lunch at a restaurant, and we realized my mom couldn't write a check to pay for the food. It broke my heart while at the same time, I realized I was going to have to take up a new role.

This new role would include not only experiencing the loss myself as a daughter, but also taking on the role as the oldest sister of looking after my sisters in a maternal way to make sure they were doing okay as well.

Another snapshot I have, is when we were thinking about moving to Michigan to plant a church and feeling God's leadership in our lives to do that. I remember asking my mom and dad what they thought and realizing how much things would change with me being far away, and not being able to help as much as I would want. And I remember my mom and dad so clearly telling me that they wouldn't want her diagnosis to stop me and my husband from responding to God's call on our lives. Making that decision to move has definitely changed my experience with mom and her Alzheimer's, because what I experience with her now is more in snapshots, rather than seeing the slow steady decline that everyone else sees. It also caused me to grieve a little more quickly because of not being able to see her as often and not being able to talk to her on the phone (since she could not really use it very well).

The loss has felt so great, and what I hate the most is that my kids haven't gotten an accurate representation of who my mom really is. When we first moved, she would still come up and stay with us for a week at a time and was always amazing with the kids and was so present with them – which was so helpful due to the challenges of me as a young busy mom. I loved that at least my older kids got that from her. As her disease progressed, she wasn't able to come by herself anymore, and then eventually she couldn't come up at all.

I have another clear memory. A couple of years ago on my kid's first day of school, when my fourth was starting kindergarten and my youngest was in preschool, I remember that night after all of the excitement and stress that day held, making sure everything was ready for all 5 kids to get off to school and the prep work that had happened. The memory was that my husband had gone for something and I was at home feeding the kids dinner by myself and I suddenly had this overwhelming grief. I recognized there was no one to check on me on that eventful day – I needed a mom to say "Hey, how did your kids' first day of school go and all the stress and all that that held?" At that moment, I recognized another way of feeling the loss, knowing that no one else but a mother knows that feeling as a mom, as to what that experience is like and can really look after a daughter in the same way that you need at that time.

I recognize now, that while there is so much loss and I hate that I don't have my mom here to ask me those questions or care for me and to let me ask her my questions, she actually is closer than I think. I had this realization a year ago that there's a lot more of my mom inside of me than I had previously recognized. I know I have her laid back yet intentional style of parenting, and her way of always creating a hospitable environment for people who come into her home. And although I don't have her to ask specific questions, I now understand that she had been training me my whole life to do this. This is what discipleship really is.

In closing this is what I realized. As you do the hard work of rearing your kids to love Jesus and walk with Him, you equip your kids to do life without you since you will not always be there. And while I would much rather have her mentally and physically with me, I am thankful that she gave me everything she had in the days she could. It shaped me to be the mom and person I am today and it is shaping those around me. So be encouraged if you are investing in others – your impact goes beyond you – when you teach them to love and serve others the way He does.

Next is from my second daughter, Amy:

My dad asked us all to reflect on mom's diagnosis and how it has affected us, while we are quarantined at home. I have so many thoughts on this, but the first thing that comes to my mind is loss. I just feel a weight of loss that is hard to describe. My mom is the best person I know, and I just feel like I lost that person too early. I feel like my kids lost the chance to know her as a grandmother. I feel like my dad lost her as an empty nest companion. I feel like Waco and the world lost one of its greatest servants too early.

I felt a lot of loss this February when my son was diagnosed with leukemia. This is when my mom would have shined. She LOVED to serve people, especially the sick, and I know she would have done everything possible to help us during this time. I love how God sees me when I am feeling the loss, and meets me there. I felt (and continue to feel) so loved and cared for by my family and friends that I didn't just stay stuck in the feelings of loss for my mom. God is so kind to us. "My grace is sufficient for you, for my power is made perfect in weakness. Therefore, I will boast all the more gladly of my weaknesses, so that the power of Christ may rest upon me." 2 Corinthians 12:9

The loss for my kids is heavy for me. They missed out on years and years of experiencing one of the sweetest grandmothers ever. I tell them stories about her and try and describe her, but it just isn't the same as them experiencing it. I love seeing parts of my mom in my kids and describing it to them. They love hearing how they are like her. I love that my kids are in the same order as my own family, so as I parent them, I can think about how mom handled it all. I do wish I could ask her for advice on parenting. I still have her old phone number saved in my phone and my heart catches when I see it there, just aching to call her and tell her a cute story Lucy did or a sweet moment with me and the kids, or how to make sure every kid feels loved and cared for! So many things I wish I could talk to her about!

Seeing my dad have to walk through his empty nest years taking care of mom has been really hard for me. I feel so much loss for him. I have been completely blown away by his ability to love and serve mom and us through this, but it just breaks my heart for him. He has lost his wife so early. I would have loved to see all the ways they would have served the Lord together in their empty nest years. I would have loved watching them babysit the grandkids together, go on mission trips, serve those around them and just love their time together after over 20 years of raising kids.

As you can see, the loss I feel is great. It has been such an interesting process for me. I will be fine for months with everything and then I will see a grandma back to school shopping with her grandkids and start crying in the mall. The grief comes in waves and you can't predict when it will hit. Putting my mom in the memory facility was one of the hardest things I have ever done, but I know it was the right thing. One of my mom's favorite words is HOPE and I am so glad that it was. I feel like even now, 12 years in, I have hope. I have hope that God can still heal her. I have hope that he is working all things for good. We all need to cling to hope, especially right now, so I am thankful she taught me that. "Now hope does not disappoint, because the love of God has been poured out in our hearts by the Holy Spirit who was given to us." Romans 5:5

Next is from my son Jason:

I have been known to be my mom's favorite. At least that's what I always told her. She would correct me and say, "Jason, you are. You are my favorite son" (which does not say much as I am the only son)! I have handled Alzheimer's differently in some ways than my sisters. I am a positive, hopeful, optimistic person. So, when mom was initially diagnosed, I had so much confidence that God would heal her or that she would stabilize and not get any worse. Well, year after year I was faced with the reality of the situation, the continued decline of my mom. I have trouble tapping into my emotions and going to painful places, so I don't want to do that for another post. If you want tears, check out my sisters' blog posts, ha.

One of the hardest parts about Alzheimer's for me is not with the person's forgetfulness, but our forgetfulness. Hmm. I'm talking about forgetting who my mom was, remembering what she was like, how she would sound, how she hugged, her laugh, her quirks. I remember her being one of my favorite people in the world. I remember her not having an enemy, loving every single person on the planet. I remember that she impacted people at our schools, church, K-Life, high school students, college students, single women, married women, etc. I know those things are true, but I forget the specifics. So, for this post, I want to share stories I do remember, ones that make me smile, and hopefully make you smile and know/or remember her a little bit more.

Perm Performance – My mom was beautiful, no doubt. For some reason though, a certain hairstyle took the 90's by storm and in which my mom was swept up, "The Perm". I remember her coming home from the salon and the stench of her hair from the perm permeating the house. I remember the tight curls in which her hair was bound. I'll be honest – I was a little embarrassed, so my response every time was to take both my hands and rub her head to try and loosen up the curls. Yikes, how annoying and immature I must have been. But she still loved and favored me. How I would love to see her come home with a perm right now and give her a big kiss on her head.

Limbaugh Lunch - When I was in 6th grade, I was homeschooled by my parents. My mom was a little laxer than my dad. Mom's method of teaching typically came through Rush Limbaugh (haha). We regularly left home for lunch around 10:30/11 to pick up a Wonton soup for my mom from Magic China and my favorite, Wendy's. I remember taking in a fair share of Rush Limbaugh while making these stops and running other errands. She loved that guy. I am not 100% sure but pretty confident I passed Mom's subjects that year with all A's, but on my dad's side (science) I received a D. How I would love to make those errands while listening to Rush with her right now.

Diet Cokes- My mom not only loved Magic China, but she loved Diet Coke. Somehow my mom made a simple Diet Coke both impactful and hilarious. She would daily visit the McDonalds on Valley Mills/Wooded Acres intersection. Over her visits, she made great friends with this one lady who worked there. When I would ride with her, it was as if these two were lifelong friends. She would ask how so and so was doing, going deeper than most drive thru' interactions. But that's who she was; she made friends wherever she went, when no one else was watching. The other local establishment she frequently visited for a Diet Coke was Wards Liquor Store. A liquor store – who would have thought? I have no clue how she found out they had great Diet Cokes because she didn't drink alcohol, but this place had become a favorite of hers. And I love that about her. How I'd love to pick her up a Diet Coke and sit on our front porch and talk with her.

Cheerleader- I remember my mom being so proud of me as a student, even though I wasn't that great of one. The SAT was a big stressor for me AND my parents. After bombing a few practice SATs, I'd say all of our confidence in the real deal was lacking. At the time, you could take the SAT, wait a couple weeks, then call in to a phone operator and receive your scores. This was a big deal for me, because with what I was getting on my practice SATs, it wasn't looking like I was getting into college. When the scores were available, mom came and sat with me on my bed while we listened to the operator. We prayed and waited eagerly for those scores. When the final score came through, she celebrated as if I had made a perfect score (and it was far from that). How I'd love for her to believe with me for something right now.

I remember the morning of my wedding; my mom and I went to breakfast. We had a tearful, wonderful conversation. I wish I had taken notes or recorded what she said. One thing I do remember was her saying, "Jas, now, if you have any questions about tonight, you know sex, you can ask me. I was like "Mom, Noooo. Never. Awkward. Why would you ask me that?" She didn't care, she was just so sweet. Her sweetness always broke any awkwardness. How I'd love for her to ask me whatever she wanted, just to have a conversation with her right now.

Friend and Comforter- One story, I hold on to dearly and may have been told before was from her trip to Haiti after the earthquake in 2010. She was only a couple years into her diagnosis, and her symptoms were mild. Our church was sending a team of first responders to care for the tens and hundreds of thousands hurt and affected by the earthquake. My mom was in. She saw a need and wanted to go. She joined the team with our friend Donny Martin. Donny shares this story so well. They were walking through the streets caring for the sick and hurting, sharing the gospel, seeing people's lives touched by God. Donny was feeling really confident until he came to one tent. A Haitian woman had lost an arm and the infection was turning really bad. Donny got ready to enter the tent, but the odor from her rotting arm was just too much, he couldn't enter the tent. He was about to vomit. It took him several minutes before he gained composure to enter the tent. He opened the flap to the tent and there sitting, embracing this woman with a missing arm was my mom. This woman's head was in my mom's chest, cradling her, singing to her. The smell of rotting flesh didn't thwart my mom from loving someone in need. That's what she would do; that's who she was. How I'd love to rest my head on her chest and hear her heart beat, for her to sing her sweet songs in my ear right now.

I remember my mom being so inclusive. People felt so comfortable around her. They trusted her and could confide in her. We always say she could sit in a room with Kings and Queens as well as the poor or the mentally handicapped and she wouldn't change a bit.

One day, God willing, I will remember more stories about my mom. For now, I tear up with faint memories of my mom. How I wish so badly to embrace her? And for her to embrace me back. To drive through Magic China listening to Rush Limbaugh. How I wish to take a nap with her. To watch her play with our kids. To love and encourage my wife. How I'd love to see her and my dad laugh together. For them both to look on with pride at their grandchildren.

And lastly, my youngest daughter, Mary Beth:

Grief. If you know anything about me you know that I am not one to shy away from big feelings, dark emotions or the like. I would rather stare a feeling straight in the face and fully experience it before it passes as time naturally allows. "This too shall pass." A common phrase you hear in the midst of difficult times as an encouragement. However, in the face of certain forms of grief – here I am... I'm still waiting... it's not passing...

Most of you probably know the different phases of grief. The wisdom that is applied in healing through times of tragedy is to let those phases take their course. I can do that. I can do that well because I struggle to leave a phase until I feel that it has been fully and authentically fulfilled. I appreciate those times of longing/anger/angst because they are real and healthy and necessary. They are an emotional response that you can see is a part of this beautiful process to heal, and not to simply bandage.

But alas, this all brings us to what this blog is about: My mom. At least to me it is about my mom, but to you I guess it is more about the long suffering of the caregiver to an Alzheimer's patient. Let's come back to the beloved quote: "This too shall pass." But with Alzheimer's it doesn't. Well not really.

I was in high school when I started noticing the changes in my mom. I was in college when she was "Diagnosed". But that was just the beginning. There were the big events in my life like meeting my husband, engagement, and our wedding where I was getting a taste of how much of my mom was missing. But that was just the beginning. Those were the early years of Alzheimer's.

Later came the grief of not having my mom be physically capable of holding my children, or to look them in their eyes, or even to call them by name. And then there came the grief of her not looking me in the eyes, her not lighting up when she heard me walk in through the door and for her not even knowing my name. In those years there were countless joys and enumerable losses. There are days now that I begin weeping while folding laundry, because the longing for my mother is so deep that it overtakes me. I remember that there were several times in my childhood when my mom would act the same way around me. She would be folding laundry in the middle of our hallway and employ me with the socks. She would begin weeping out of nowhere and when I asked her why she was crying, all she would say was: "I miss my mom." In those times my mom was over a decade past the loss of her mom (at age 62 of lung cancer before I was even born and my mother was 32), so I struggled to understand what could cause these sudden outbursts of grief. I understand now. Grief is unsettling. There is no timeline, and maybe there never is a timeline. And then with Alzheimer's there is no "six months to a year." There are constant losses and another wave of greater losses topped with the hard decisions.... And yet they– the ones we love/desire/long for– are still here.

I remember the day my mom left after staying and helping us for a few weeks after we had our first baby. She couldn't drive at the point so my aunt came up to Dallas to drive her back home. I remember us weeping in the entryway of my home as we grieved the loss of that special time together. That moment will be grafted into my memory as one of so many unspoken words, but of a beautiful closure. We both recognized that there was something more to that moment. It would be the last time that she was able to truly help. She knew she was seeing that she was leaving me more than just that physical moment. But it was prophetic of what was to come— her baby was now a new mom holding her own baby with the fear and the cry of "how do I do this without you??" And that call would be ringing out of me even as my babies grow, as it did for her decades after the loss of her own mother.

In all honesty and utter vulnerability, I am trying to understand how I can prepare myself for the final "loss" and the grief that will come at that time. Just as I never want to resent the losses over the past thirteen years, but to savor the joys, because I knew it would get worse— how do you do that now? I laugh as I close this, because I am giving you no encouragement, but just my sad remembrances and my daily grievances. So, maybe I should leave you with this: When my three-year-old or five-year-old throws a fit, I encourage them to tell me as many things that they are thankful for according to their age (3 things or 5 things). Do that for yourself. Remember and be thankful. In remembering we are not forgetting the hardships but we are recognizing them and giving them their proper place. And in thanksgiving, we are taking our next step in a state of hope. Grief is present and may always be lurking, because it will, I believe, always come in waves. But let us choose thankfulness as an honor to our loved one's life. Together, let us feel the physical, emotional, and spiritual relief that comes as we choose thankfulness.

Continuing the Journey
2021

This is the last chapter, but it is not the last chapter of our story. How long it will go on, nobody knows. I will continue to travel this journey into the unknown. But before I conclude, I have some final thoughts.

The year 2020 did come to a close, but 2021 did not start out much better. For me, it began with Covid. Literally, I got tested on New Years Day, and spent the first 10 days of the year in quarantine. Fortunately, I was only sick for about 4-5 days and then I was well and had no ill after effects. I did get my Covid vaccine as well. Then a month later, the big freeze hit Texas like nothing any of us had ever seen before. I lost power for two days but did not lose water and did not have any pipes burst. I also have a wood burning fireplace in my bedroom, so I kept it going all day and night. It helped a little – for about 5-8 feet around the fireplace. The downstairs stayed around 43 degrees, but the upstairs was under 40. Certainly, I fared better than many.

In general, Covid infections have been going down, and most of the businesses are opening up and most are no longer requiring masks. The memory care facility is also opening up and I can visit anytime I want (with a mask). I have been going every day as she has an ulcer on her left ankle that will not heal, and I have been doing daily dressing changes. Covid did go through the facility back in the fall and wiped out about half of the residents on her wing (of 18 patients). The facility has recovered and her wing is almost completely full again. Unfortunately, there is no shortage of dementia patients.

On that front, it is certainly distressing that there has been so little progress made in treatments for Alzheimer's. The last new drug for it came out almost 20 years ago, and neither of the two types of medications with indications for the disease are particularly helpful. They have made strides in earlier and better detection. Part of this is due to the ADNI study of which Luana was a part many years ago. In fact, now the earliest signs on a PET scan can be seen some 15-25 years before the onset of symptoms. This will be helpful to be able to treat earlier if any new meds do come out.

For the past few months, our family has our smart phone alarms set for 1:03 pm and it is from Psalm 103 where, especially in verse 3, the psalmist speaks of God who heals all of our diseases. So, we all stop and pray for Luana. Our prayer is that she would be healed from this horrible disease. But if not healed here on this earth, our prayer is that He would take her to be with Him in heaven, where she would be healed completely. I am okay with either way on that. In fact, when I go see her now, there is a real dichotomy in my feelings. On the one hand, it really is good to see her, even in her condition. On the other hand, I walk away from there depressed every time, seeing her in that state and knowing that she would hate being like that.

So, where do we go from here? There is no indication that she is going to pass anytime soon. She is still very healthy physically. She still eats very well, albeit slowly, and does not seem to aspirate, though she has to be fed every bite. She did lose about 20 pounds early in the course of the disease, but over the past year or more, her weight has been stable. We are somewhere between 13-15 years into her disease, where the average lifespan is only 7-11 years. She could go any day, or she could live another 8-10 years. The thought of that makes me tremble. I have no desire for her to continue to live like she is now. I know for sure that she would not. She is a DNR and I do not do anything to keep her alive, other than the basics of food and water. But she never seems to get sick.

As for me, I plan to work about four more years (till age 70), and then what? Will I be able to afford the memory care facility? Will I try to take her back home then? There are so many questions – and so few answers. Even though I have seen a lot of what this journey has to offer, there is still a lot that remains unknown. I have no choice but to continue to travel down this road.

My goal in writing this book was not to give more information on Alzheimer's. There are plenty of books on that. It was not even meant to be a source of help for caregivers, though certainly there is plenty of that in the book – and even more on my blog. The real goal was to show the faithfulness of God – both in preparing us for the journey, and to walk with us every step of the way. I tried to show that events in our lives and our disciplined approach to following Him, gave us the confidence to trust Him to be faithful in this new struggle. And I hope I was able to convey that God has been gracious and faithful to me through every stage, to give me what I needed at the time. I never felt alone or abandoned. He was also gracious to Luana in that He gave her the courage to live life as normal as possible for as long as she could, and the peace to handle the fears that confronted her daily.

Through reading this, I pray that your faith will be encouraged to trust God in whatever challenges you will inevitably face. He is worthy of our trust.

Acknowledgements

As with any book, this was not a one person show. I first have to thank my wife, Luana, the unwitting main character in the book. She always wanted me to write a book, and even went so far as to buy me a book on how to write a book. She would be embarrassed and angry that my book was about her, but still proud that I did it. She has always been my biggest cheerleader. I am just sad that she never got to see the finished product. In addition, I have to give a big thanks to my four children. Not only have they been so helpful to me in taking care of Luana, and have experienced the devastation of the disease firsthand, but have been so encouraging in my writing. They have given me good critiques as to the content as well. I have to give thanks to my friend, Annette Perez, an old English teacher, who did an amazing and careful job of the grammatical editing. Then there is Micah Key who did the content editing and graphic design and provided plenty of advice along the way.

About the Author

This is the first book by Arthur Sudan, M.D. His day job is as an internist in Waco, Texas, where he has been practicing for the past 36 years. He has been married to Luana for 44 years and has four children and sixteen grandchildren. He graduated from Baylor University and Baylor College of Medicine and he continues to be an avid Bears' fan. His other hobbies include playing tennis, hiking, gardening, woodworking, photography and reading. In addition, for ten years he was an adjunct professor of biology at Baylor University, teaching on aging. He is an active member and lifegroup leader at Antioch Community Church in Waco.

About the Book

Journey Into The Unknown is a story about Alzheimer's disease, but even more so, it is a story about the faithfulness of God in the difficult times of life. Artie Sudan is a physician in Internal Medicine who has taken care of hundreds, if not thousands of patients with Alzheimer's. He has given out much advice to their caregivers and would consider himself an expert in the field.

But when his own wife is diagnosed with early onset Alzheimer's disease at age 53, he begins a journey into unknown territory – being a caregiver himself. He finds that all of his advice and experience over the years, while good, did not prepare him for all that this new job would require. This job takes him totally out of his comfort zone and beyond his giftings. But he is not without resources and he does not give in to despair.

This book also traces a long line of God's faithfulness to Artie and his wife, Luana, over the decades before this dreaded diagnosis. He describes how each of these instances become like little stones of remembrances that he puts in his altar to God where he worships. This then becomes a well from which he draws when he needs the strength to go on or to handle a new situation.

This is a story about a real person, with real struggles, doubts and questions. It does not make him out to be a super saint. It does show God to be super, but even more so, to be faithful. As you read their story, you will be encouraged that you, too, can rely on the faithfulness of God when you encounter your own journeys into the unknown.

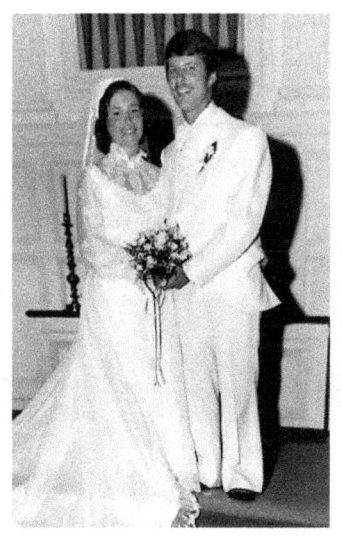
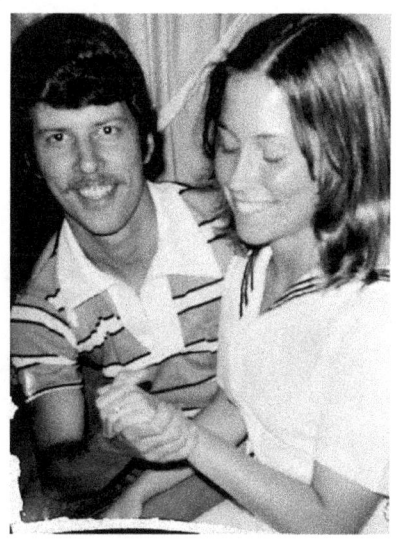
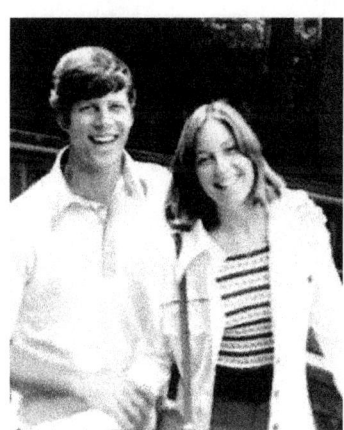
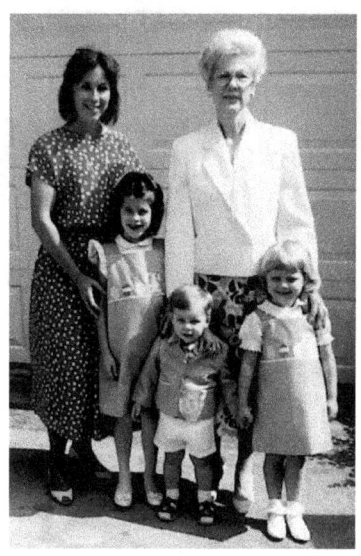

Clockwise from top left: Our wedding, 1977; Engagement Day, 1976; Luana with my mother and our early family, 1987; Early days of courtship, 1977.

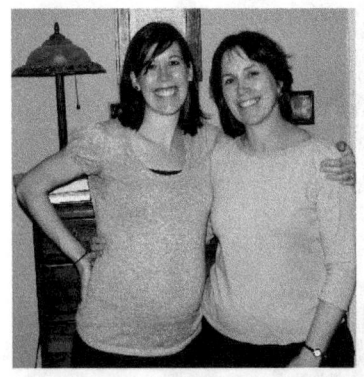
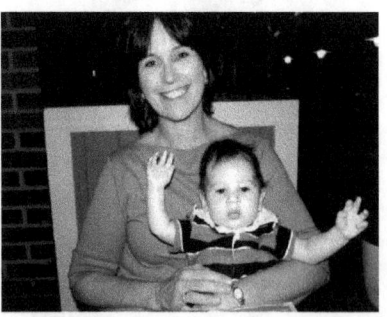
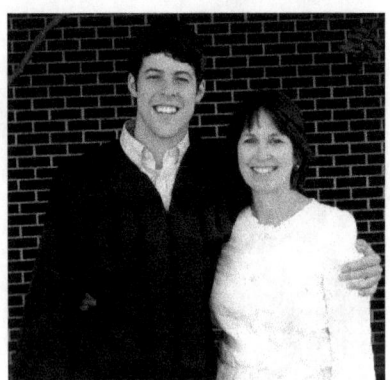
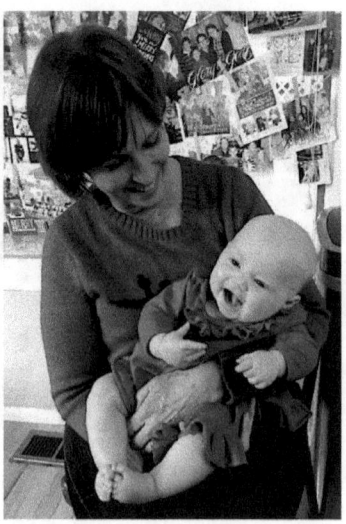

Clockwise, from top left. Luana with Christy, pregnant 2007; Luana with Jayden 2008; Luana with Lucy, 2015; Luana with Jason, graduation, 2003

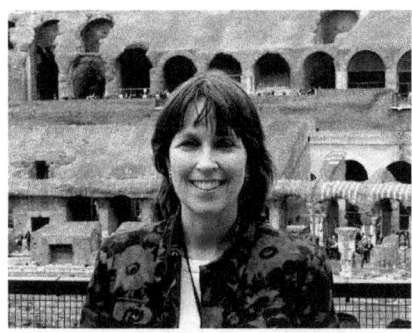
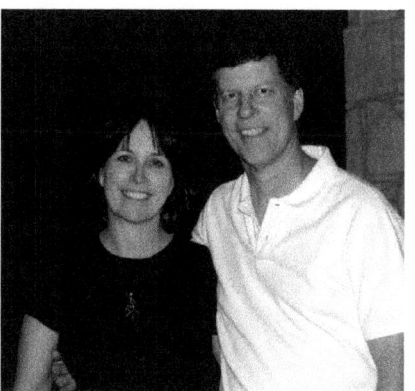
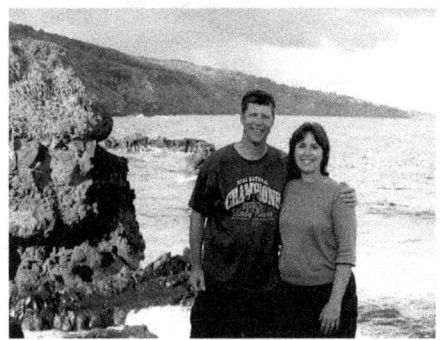
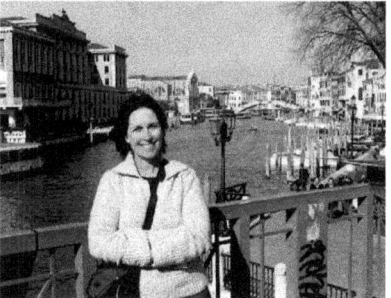

Clockwise, from top left: Luana in Rome, 2009; Luana and me, circa 2005; Luana in Venice, 2013; Luana and me in Hawaii, 2006.

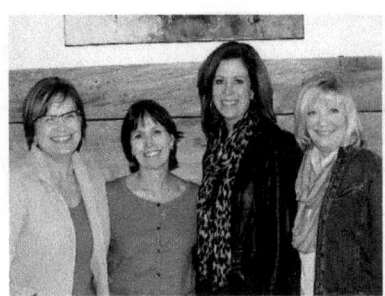
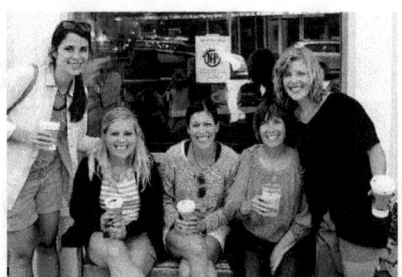
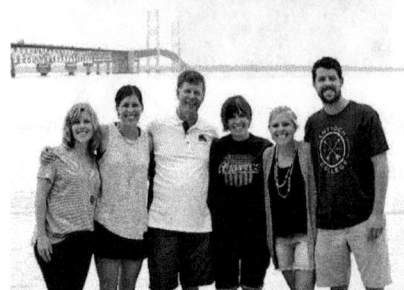
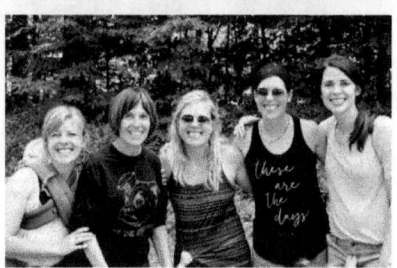

Clockwise from top left: Luana with her three faithful high school friends; Luana and the girls in Michigan, 2017; Luana and the girls on a hike, 2015; the family in Michigan, 2017.

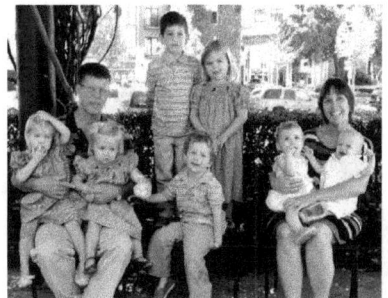
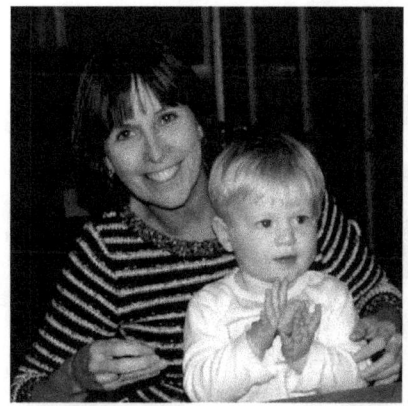
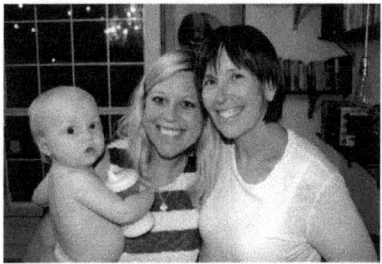
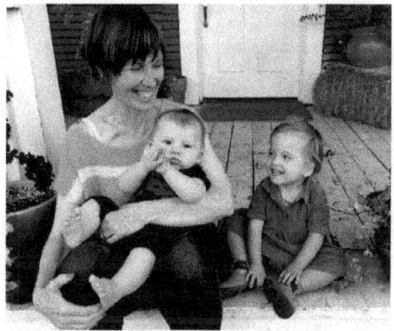

Clockwise from top left: Luana and me with our first seven grandchildren, 2012; Luana with Burson, 2016; Luana with Sunny and Sylvin, 2017; Luana with Amy and Lucy, 2015.

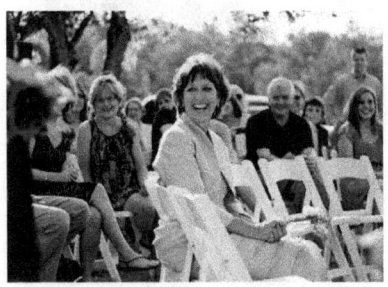
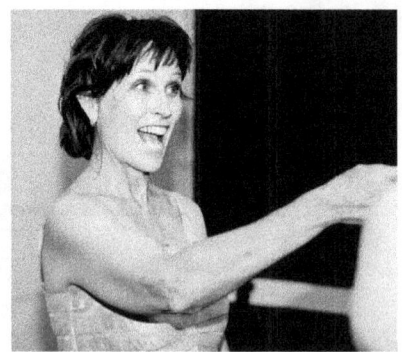
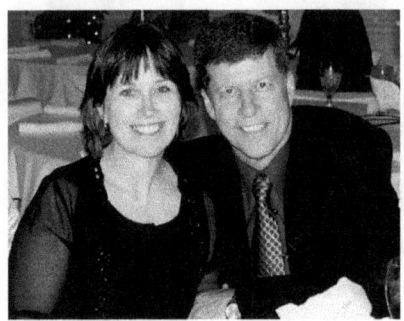
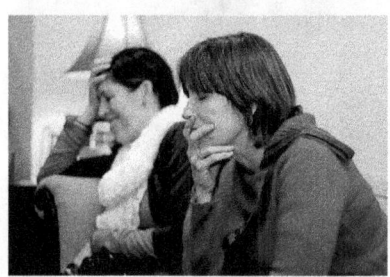

Clockwise from top left: Luana at Mary Beth's wedding, 2012; Luana dancing at same wedding; Luana in prayer; Luana and me at a friend's wedding.

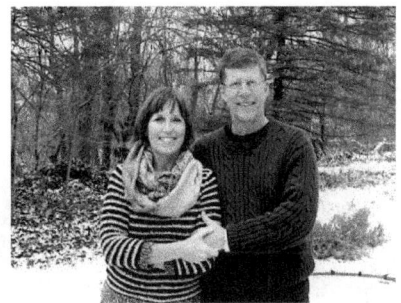
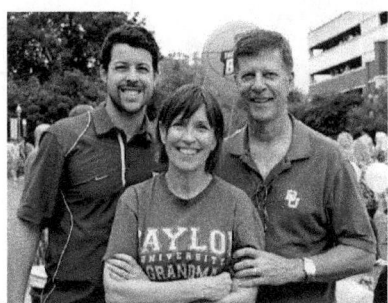
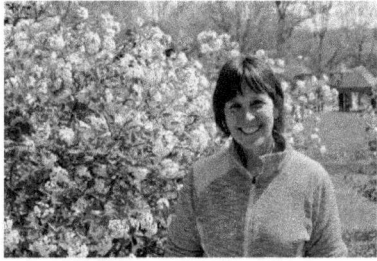

Clockwise from top left: Luana and me at Thanksgiving in Michigan, 2013; Luana in Michigan in Spring, 2016; Luana, me and Jason at Baylor Homecoming, 2016.

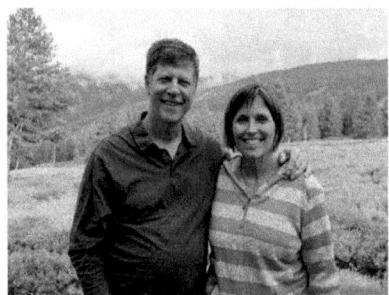
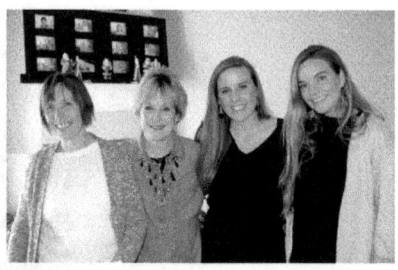
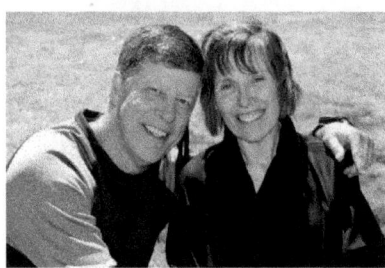
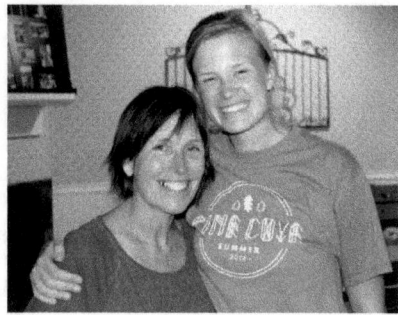

Clockwise from top left: Luana and me in Colorado, 2016; Luana with her sister and nieces, Stephanie and Anna Lee at Christmas, 2017; Luana with Kristen, 2016; Luana and me, 2019.

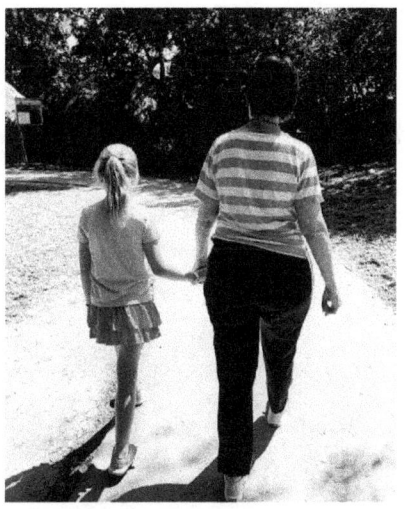
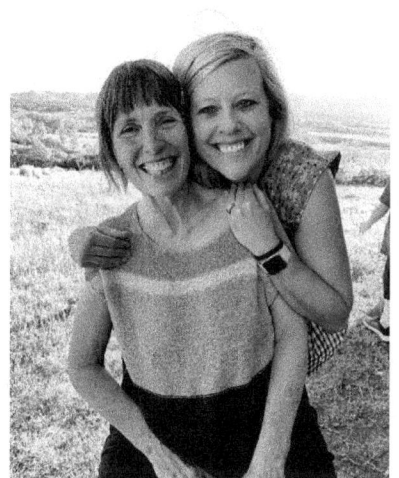
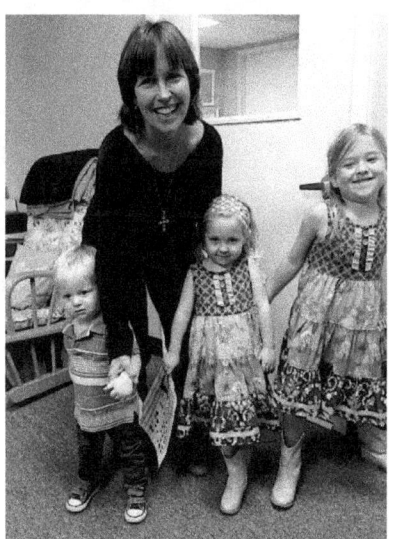
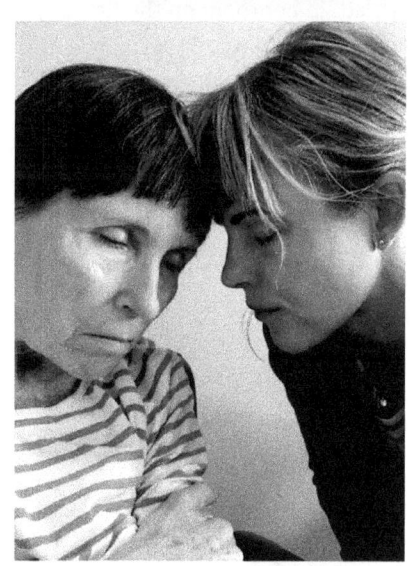

Clockwise from top left: Emery Kate leading Luana by the hand as she often did, 2018; Amy with Luana, 2019; Mary Beth with Luana in prayer and anguish, 2021; Luana with the Marable kids, 2014.

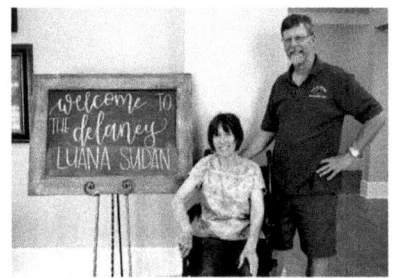
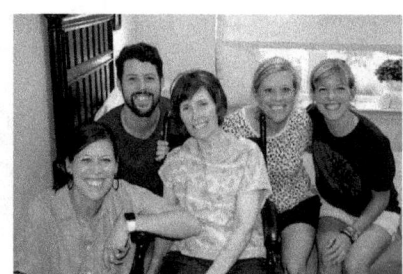
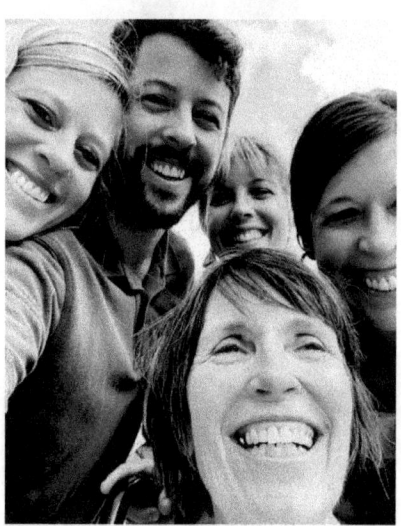

Clockwise from top left: Luana as she enters the memory care facility, 2019; Luana and the kids in her room on the first day at the facility, 2019; Luana and the kids in a selfie at the facility, 2019; Our whole family in Colorado, 2019.

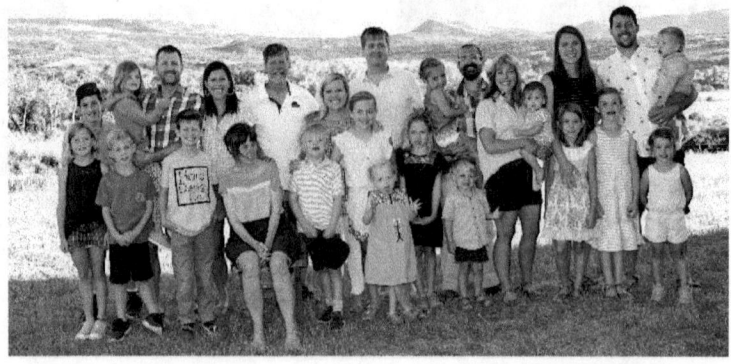

www.ingramcontent.com/pod-product-compliance
Lightning Source LLC
Chambersburg PA
CBHW070916030426
42336CB00014BA/2431